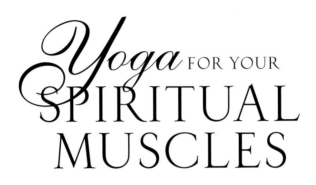

Yoga FOR YOUR
SPIRITUAL
MUSCLES

Praise for
YOGA FOR YOUR SPIRITUAL MUSCLES

"What more could you want in a yoga book? Wonderful exercises for your body, mind, emotions, and spirit. Powerful spiritual principles you can use in your everyday life. Postures, breathing, and meditations to reinforce what you've learned. You will find your physical muscles stretched, your mind inspired, your heart opened up, and your spiritual self nourished."

—Judi Neal, Ph.D., Associate Professor, Center for Spirit at Work, University of New Haven

"A deeply joyful way to strengthen and energize your spirit while stretching and toning your body. Rachel's imaginative approach to spiritual yoga is much like my own. I am delighted to see this book."

—Lilias Folan, author, international yoga teacher, and host of the yoga video series *Lilias*

"I can think of no better person than Rachel Schaeffer to help me find and flex my spiritual muscles. She is one of those rare teachers who embodies what she teaches: compassion, acceptance, patience, and strength. She embues her love of yoga with a healthy dose of playfulness and laughter—a lesson for all of us who take life too seriously."

—Linda Sparrowe, contributing editor and former managing editor of *Yoga Journal*

"Rachel Schaeffer truly makes yoga accessible to the Western mind, body, and spirit. Her approach is both practical and timeless, challenging and user friendly. The idea that we can create our own postures to develop our own spiritual muscles is revolutionary and timely. Don't miss this book!"

—Christine Caldwell, Ph.D., author of *Getting in Touch: The Guide to New Body-Centered Therapies*

"Rachel's conversational tone is comforting, inspiring, and reassuring. The way she blends everyday situations like work stress with her sense of humor makes me want to return again and again. A delight to read and a must have for wellness professionals."

—Ruth M. Warren, Associate Director, Program Development, The Fisher Institute of Wellness, Ball State University

"A remarkable contribution to the growing body of yoga literature. Clear instruction, interesting text, and inspiring delivery. An enduring yoga book, full of insight, practical applications of ancient practices, and fun."

—Amy Kline Gage, President Emeritus, International Association of Yoga Therapists

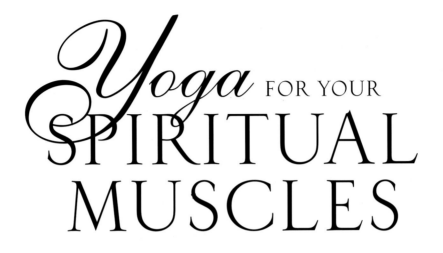

Yoga FOR YOUR SPIRITUAL MUSCLES

A Complete Yoga Program to Strengthen Body and Spirit

RACHEL SCHAEFFER

Photographs by Adam Mastoon and David S. Waitz

A publication supported by
THE KERN FOUNDATION

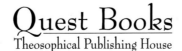

Theosophical Publishing House

Wheaton, Illinois ◆ Chennai (Madras), India

DEDICATION

To the three most important people in my life: my husband and my parents. I count as my greatest blessing that the three of you are in my life.

The Theosophical Publishing House
P.O. Box 270
Wheaton, IL 60189-0270

A publication of the Theosophical Publishing House,
a department of the Theosophical Society in America

Grateful thanks to Donna Karan and her staff for the use of DKNY clothing for the author and the models.

Cover and text design and typesetting by Beth Hansen-Winter

Library of Congress Cataloging-in-Publication Data

Schaeffer, Rachel.
Yoga for your spiritual muscles: a complete yoga program to strengthen body and spirit / Rachel Schaeffer;
photographs by Adam Mastoon and David S. Waitz. — 1st Quest ed.
p.   cm.
ISBN 0-8356-0763-1

1. Yoga, Hatha.   I. Mastoon, Adam.   II. Waitz, David S.   III. Title.
RA781.7.S295   1998
613.7'046—dc21   97-41048
                                                            CIP

Printed in Hong Kong through Global Interprint, Petaluma, California

6   5   4   3   2   *   98   99   00   01   02   03

Grateful acknowledgment is made for permission to reprint copyrighted material: Reprinted from *Being Peace* (1987) by Thich Nhat Hanh with permission of Parallax Press, Berkeley, CA. Leon Shenandoah-Six Nations Iroquois Confederacy ©1990 Steve Wall and Harvey Arden, from the book *Wisdomkeepers*, Beyond Words Publishing, Inc., 1-800-284-9673. From *Start Where You Are* by Pema Chodron ©1994. Reprinted by arrangement with Shambhala Publications Inc., 300 Massachusetts Ave., Boston, MA 02115. From *Man's Eternal Quest* by Paramahansa Yogananda, Self-Realization Fellowship (Los Angeles, 1982). B.K.S. Iyengar, *Light On Yoga* ©1966, Schocken Books. "Chant for Self-Esteem" from *Jamabalaya: The Natural Woman's Book of Personal Charms and Practical Rituals* by Luisah Teish, copyright ©1985 by Luisah Teish. Reprinted by permission of HarperCollins Pub., Inc. Excerpt as submitted from *A Return to Love* by Marianne Williamson, copyright ©1992 by Marianne Williamson. Reprinted by permission of HarperCollins Pub., Inc., portions reprinted from *A Course in Miracles*, copyright ©1975 by Foundation for Inner Peace, Inc. All chapter openings are from *A Course in Miracles*. From *A Path with Heart*, Jack Kornfield, Bantam Books. From *The Essence of Tai Chi Ch'uan—The Literary Tradition* by Lo, Inn, Amacker, and Foe, copyright ©1979 by Benjamin Pang Jeng Lo, Martin Inn, Susan Foe, and Robert Amacker. Reprinted with permission of North Atlantic Books, P.O.Box 12327, Berkeley, CA 94710. Reprinted from *Breathe! You're Alive: Sutra on the Full Awareness of Breathing* (1996) by Thich Nhat Hanh with permission of Parallax Press, Berkeley, CA. From *Shambhala: The Sacred Path of the Warrior* by Chogyam Trungpa ©1984. Reprinted by arrangement with Shambhala Publications Inc., 300 Massachusetts Ave., Boston, MA 02115. From *Full Catastrophe Living: Using the Wisdom of Your Body and Mind to Face Stress, Pain, and Illness*, Jon Kabat-Zinn, Delta. Excerpt as submitted from *The Essential Tao*, translated and presented by Thomas Cleary, copyright ©1991 by Thomas Cleary. Reprinted by permission of HarperCollins Pub., Inc. From *Beyond Words* by Sri Swami Satchidananda, copyright ©1977 by Satchidananda Ashram-Yogaville. Reprinted by permission of Satchidananda Ashram-Yogaville. From *Zen Mind, Beginners Mind* by Shunryu Suzuki, ©1973 John Weatherhill Inc. From *The Quiet Mind*, White Eagle, ©1972 White Eagle Publishing Trust. From *Meditations* by Marcus Aurelius, translated by Maxwell Staniforth, Great Britain 1986, p. 115, ©Maxwell Staniforth 1964. Reproduced by permission of Penguin Books, Ltd. From *Emmanuel's Book*, compilers Pat Rodegast & Judith Stanton, Bantam Books.

ACKNOWLEDGMENTS

To quote singer/songwriter David Roth, my deep gratitude to "the Unseen Hands that guide us and the miracles that cause us to believe." There are so many special people who have directly and indirectly contributed to this book. Please forgive me if I have inadvertently left any one out.

Heartfelt appreciation to Brenda Rosen, who graciously helped my dream become a reality, and all the folks at Quest Books including Sharron Dorr, Kim Oakley, Nancy Grace, and Vija Bremanis. To Beth Hansen Winter, whose book design graces the eyes of all who witness it. Thanks to Sandi Kazmeir for the spectacular colorization of my reflection on the front cover. To Jane Lawrence, my copy editor who generously shared her story of healing as she meticulously went through each piece of the book. To the staff at *Yoga Journal*: Linda Sparrowe, Jennifer Barrett, Ron Alexander, Steve O'Rourke. Your early support and warm hearts helped to light my way.

My gratitude to the delightful and talented people at Donna Karan International: Donna herself for the generous use of her incredibly comfortable and elegant yoga/fitness clothes, Patti Cohen, Stacey Berger, Cindy Capobianco, Dina Columbo, and Vernon Yenick. To the generous and wonderful people at the Pleasantdale Chateau: Wade Knowles and family, Christopher Gellings, Sylvia Calabrese, and Mary Jane Frankel.

My sincere love and thanks to all of my students at Montclair State University and Caldwell College —you have all been my teachers. To all of my colleagues at Caldwell College and Montclair State University, especially Tim Sullivan, Rob Gilbert, and Susan Schwager.

To Adam Mastoon and David S. Waitz, you guys are not only talented and professional wizards, but also dear and fun friends who maintained your sense of humor throughout incredibly long days (and nights), bad take-out food, and other hilarious adventures suitable for "Saturday Night Live." Enormous thanks to the dedicated models, who came from near and far and cheerfully endured long hours of posture holding: Alicia Scott, Juliarose Loffredo, Ian Magpantay, Madeleine Weinreich, Ann Greene, Todd Norian, and Elly Gardner. Special thanks to Stephen Cope: I can't imagine what my life would have been like without your beautiful friendship. Thanks and hugs to the "Yoga Story" people who shared their stories with honesty and brilliant humanness: Lynne Davies, Kris Jacobsen, Leslie Simmons, Jonji Provenzano (and Debra Provenzano of The Yoga Studio in Kingston, NY), Bernice Lewis, Jeff Migdow, Anamika Coleman, Nateshvar Ken Scott, Jaganath Carrera, David Gershon, Gail Straub, and Stephen Cope. Special thanks to Morris Rubin, who at this writing is about to celebrate his 97th birthday: you are an inspiration!

To all teachers in the lineages of every yogic tradition—thank you for preserving this most precious gift. To the folks who made and make Kripalu Center what it is, especially my yoga teachers: Christopher Baxter, Megha (Nancy Foust) who I am proud to call my twin yoga sister, Deva Parnell, Rudy Peirce, Patricia Niti Seip, Jayvadan Howard Schwartzberg. To the folks who called me "the baby" of our Yoga Teacher Training: I loved having you all as my family! Thanks to Cynthia Casterella (Gayatri) my beloved first yoga teacher, Sarah Hartigan, Nina Manolson, Laurie Moon, Sandra Scherer (Dayashakti), Atma Jo Ann Levitt, Bhavani Lorraine Nelson, Mary Stout (Premshakti), Lucinda Hudson, Michael Lee, Mark Kapner (Ashvin),

Sigitas Baltramaitis (Yatish), Trupti, and Elaine Beaufait at the Kripalu Yoga Teacher Association.

Thanks to John Reeser and Lois Hazel at Rodale Books for your enthusiasm and friendship. Millions of twinkles to my Empowerment friends. The folks at the Fisher Institute for Wellness, especially Ruth Warren and Debbie Sheller. Richard Gonzalez, Afro-Cuban and Caribbean Dance teacher dynamo whose classes helped me get back to myself after my miscarriage. Professor Lynn Brooks and Professor Thomas Hopkins at Franklin & Marshall College, who encouraged me to practice yoga and to be my own guide. Linni Silberman-Deihl and Bob Fulrodt, for more than just professional training. My Australian friends with wise and wonderful spirits especially Margaret Scrymgour, Alan Bowker, Lu Parbery, Betti Knott, and John Henderson. Elaine Criscione, a rare and special friend and photographer whose spirit blesses everyone who meets her. With love to Jane Fried who turned me on to Shakti Gawain (thanks Shakti), and who during my decision to become a yoga teacher said "Just do it already!" In memory of Sylvia Klein Olkin, whose friendship and amazing dedication to the health of pregnant women lives on.

Thanks to my sister, Dara, we've progressed joyfully from sibling rivalry to revelry, her husband Bill, and all of my sisters and brothers-in-law, John, Madelyn, Chris, and Maryann. I am lucky to have married into such a wonderful family. To my parents-in-law, Fran and Jim, you are exceptional people and I treasure you both. To all of my precious nephews and nieces, particularly Jamie, who is my #1 role model for silliness and reminds me that fun is the first ingredient to a good life. To my grandparents for giving me the greatest gift of all: your truly unconditional love. Obbie and Grandma,

I miss you enormously. Your contribution to my life is invaluable.

My love and gratitude to my eternal friends Carrie McGuire Jones, (what in the world would I do without you?), Peg Shannon, Paula and Dan Coughlin. Corey and Suzanne Weiss, dear friends and cheerleaders extraordinaire. With deep love to Yamuna Van Looveran whose love has enriched my entire being. Kokila Gina Mazer (my creative brainstorming partner whose contribution to this book and my life are immeasurable) and her delightful parents. Special thanks to Jill Pfefer, Debbie and Jace McKeighan, Beth Gidman, Joan Anderson, Dan and Elise Blatt, Brad Pollack, Kerry Chandler, Jeannie Carter, Mirja Adams, Rick Hornung, and Peg Palmer. I am surely rich with wonderful friends.

Thanks could never be enough for my mom and dad, Michele and Michael Palmer, and my husband, Jim Schaeffer. It is impossible for me to express my profound gratitude to you three people who are the very center of my life. I have always known that I am the luckiest person in the world: I am blessed with parents whose love for me (and mine for them) has always been the solid ground on which I walk. This book, not to mention my life, could never have been possible without your unflagging support on every imaginable level.

Jim, my deepest wish to find the most spectacular companion through life's journey has been answered. From Art Director to photographic assistant, from listening patiently to every gory detail of this book's process to financial support—your name should be on the cover of this book for much of the organization and significant artistic decisions. You are a creative genius! I am healed and transformed by our love.

CONTENTS

AUTHOR'S PREFACE

This book was truly a labor of love. In fact, it was the labor I didn't have. About two years ago, my husband and I lost a baby through miscarriage. This loss runs deep and on many levels.

Prompted by my fantastic students, I became "pregnant" with this book. It helped me to integrate the experience of loss in a productive and constructive way. It's not that I replaced the baby with this book. Rather, I used the book as an opportunity to explore the multifaceted emotional landscape of my life experiences. The depth of my relationship with each of the twelve Spiritual Muscles transformed me through each stage of my "pregnancy." I nurtured *Yoga for Your Spiritual Muscles* in the womb of my heart. This literary pregnancy had its share of worries, discomforts, ecstasies, sacrifices—and even labor pains!

I'm sure that for my husband it was somewhat like living with a pregnant woman. On some days I brimmed with expectation; on others I wallowed in fatigue. Aside from my invaluable family and friends, writing helped me find the missing pages of my life that I feared I had lost. I am overwhelmed with gratitude for the large community of people that supported me and helped to midwife this act of creation. And even though it took longer than the usual forty-week gestation, I hope you will find it worthwhile, inspirational, and most importantly, practical.

As I deliver this book into the world, my sincere prayer is that it blesses those of you who let it into your lives. May *Spiritual Muscles* coach you as you enter into the ancient and healing world of yoga.

Please feel free to write to me with your own yoga story or comments: Rachel Schaeffer c/o Quest Books/ PO Box 270/ Wheaton, Illinois 60189. I would be delighted and honored to hear from you.

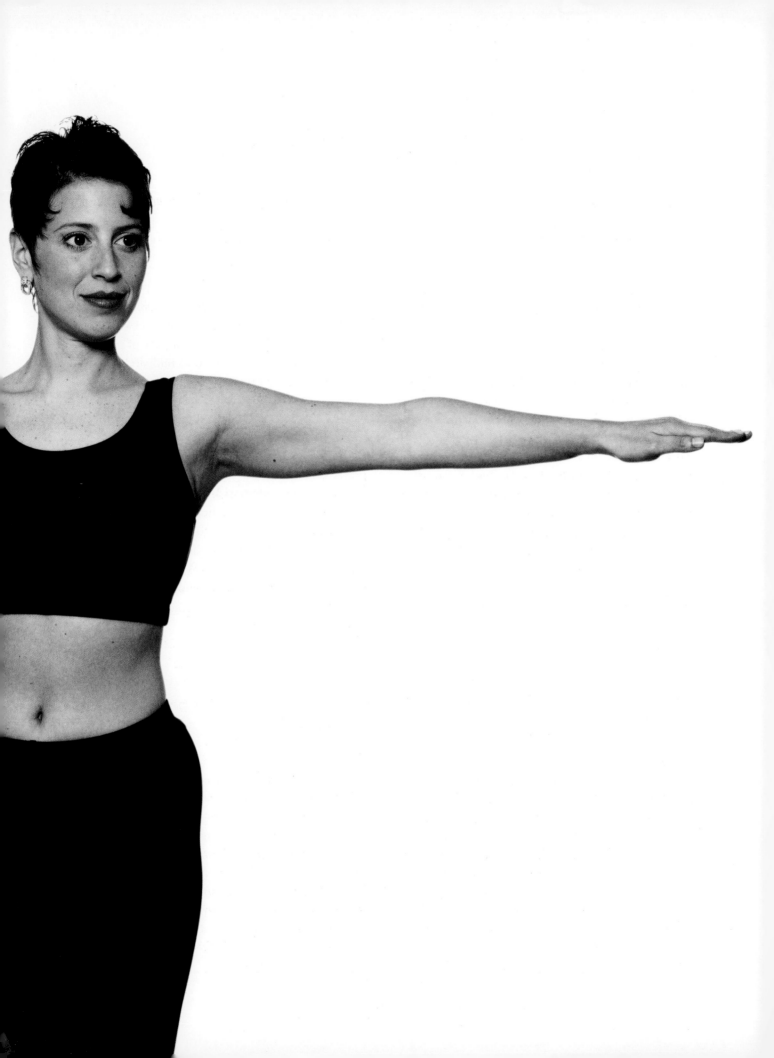

WHAT ARE SPIRITUAL MUSCLES?

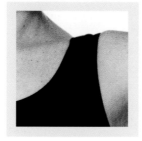

When I was at Kripalu Center training to be a yoga teacher, I kept a journal in which I recorded changes that I noticed in myself. I began the journal noting that the original reason I came to yoga was to feel better physically and to reduce stress. In truth—and what I quickly discovered—was that I was really seeking spiritual nourishment.

I described the ways in which my body was getting stronger and more flexible. But, more importantly, I observed that the spiritual parts of my being were also developing. As I was able to accept my body's limitations in a yoga posture, I was better able to accept whatever life presented to me. As I learned to breathe through challenging postures, I felt more at ease breathing through difficult decisions. When I practiced compassion with myself on days I struggled with yoga, I became a more compassionate friend to others. Whatever was happening on the yoga mat was happening off the mat. As I grounded myself in the physical, I opened my vessel for spirit to enter. Yoga strengthened my inner core, the most essential part of who I am.

Yoga had become a metaphor for my life. I felt more complete, a whole being, rather than just a body with a mind. No therapy, exercise, or other art form had ever filled my spiritual cup to overflowing as yoga did.

At first, I thought that developing life-enhancing qualities was simply a beneficial by-product of yoga. I later realized that I could *consciously* develop a *particular* inner quality, or what I have come to call a *Spiritual Muscle*. Practicing specific postures, breathing, and relaxation techniques, I discovered a way to nurture specific sacred inner treasures. I found that which I had never lost.

We all have the inherent capacity for Spiritual Muscles. Like our physical muscles, we must strengthen and tone our Spiritual Muscles so that they do not atrophy. Each time we practice a yoga posture, we create a new opportunity to be infused with spirit. The postures are mirrors for whatever needs to be seen in the moment. Yoga is a tangible ritual that offers us a sense of the intangible.

The Spiritual Muscles that were recurrent themes in my journal compose the twelve chapters of this book: Awareness, Acceptance, Focus, Flexibility, Balance, Confidence, Peace, Strength, Compassion, Energy, Playfulness, and Connectedness. The postures give structure to that which is structureless. The breath is the passageway through which spirit flows. Creating our own postures allows us to be guided by spirit. The relaxations, visualizations, and meditations redesign our mental landscapes toward our highest potential. Yoga provides the form in which spirit lives.

HOW TO USE THIS BOOK

Yoga for Your Spiritual Muscles is a classic book that you can return to time and time again at any stage in your life. Because it is organized by spiritual qualities (or muscles), you do not need to follow this book in a systematic order. You may choose one of the twelve Spiritual Muscles to focus on for a designated period of time, such as a week or a month. Allow yourself to embody on every level the quality that you choose—physical, mental, emotional, and spiritual. *Be* the quality that you wish to develop. *See* it in your daily life. Look for it in usual and not-so-usual places. Act as if you have already won the Olympic Gold Medal in Confidence, Playfulness, or whichever quality you choose.

Part and parcel of developing a particular quality is that its exact opposite often arises. This experience is similar to when you are trying not to eat a certain food, like sugar. Suddenly, everything around you is made of sugar. The same is true when you are working with the inner mysteries. Take Balance for instance. When I was writing the Balance chapter, I became more and more aware of how *out* of Balance I felt. This is perfectly normal and indicates a fine tuning of your Awareness skills. It is similar to standing in sunshine—the brighter the light, the stronger the shadow cast behind you.

As you build your Spiritual Muscles, you will also notice that they are all deeply interconnected. You must Focus to Balance. You need Confidence and Strength in order to have Compassion. Connectedness leads to Acceptance. Know that whatever Spiritual Muscle you choose, they are all beads on the same necklace.

Read the remaining introductory minichapters first. Then, before you practice any of the techniques, read each chapter through in its entirety. Developing a beautiful piece of pottery requires four elements: earth (clay) combined with air, water, and finally fire. Developing any of the Spiritual Muscles combines the postures (earth) with breathing (air) and deep relaxation (water). When you come to this point you are ready to fire the piece and discover its unique form. That final step is creating your own posture. Each chapter in *Yoga for Your Spiritual Muscles* is organized by these four elements.

At various times in your life, you may need to invoke different Spiritual Muscles. Scattered throughout, five minisections offer guidance through some of the cycles of life. *Sharing Yoga with Your Unborn Baby* provides do's and don'ts for the expectant mom. *Connect with Kids Through Yoga* shares a playful approach to bringing children into the magical world of yoga. *College Pressures: Yoga, Take Me Away!* helps students put homework, reports, and exams into perspective. *Balance Your Workday and Build Productivity on the Job* offers simple but effective ideas to incorporate yoga into the work environment. *It's Never Too Late: Yoga into Your 100s* encourages ability and agility throughout the life span. Every chapter contains an inspiring real-life excerpt, called a *Yoga Story,* to show how one or more individuals embraced yoga to strengthen a particular spiritual quality. At each stage in this adventure called life, you have the opportunity to deepen your spiritual connection.

Whatever chapter you choose, remember to remain lighthearted. Developing sacred qualities within yourself is not a chore. It is a gift.

ABOUT THE POSTURES

Yoga invites you to move your body in new ways to give every part of you, from the facial cells to the digestive system, the gift of movement. Your job is to listen to your body's messages as you flex, move, bend, and twist. Some days you will feel looser and freer than others. That is to be expected. Commit yourself to experiencing more than just the three habitual postures that many folks have limited themselves to: sitting (in a car or an office chair), standing (this includes walking to your car from sitting in your chair), and lying down (in bed so you can get up and do it all over again!).

Pay attention to your internal and external experiences as you move through the postures. You may awaken memories stored in your body. Images, colors, sounds, and pictures from your past may surface. Feelings can also arise. Often they provide important messages you need to hear. Don't be surprised if you cry, laugh, or get angry during a posture. Allow the emotion to surface and try to breathe through it. It will pass—often as quickly as it came.

The postures are designed to be practiced in a specific order, but if it doesn't work for you, create your own. Go at your own pace. Listen to the rhythm of your body, your breathing, and your inner guidance. Move slowly. Hold each posture to your personal toleration level. Pause after each posture, taking the time to integrate and to receive the benefits.

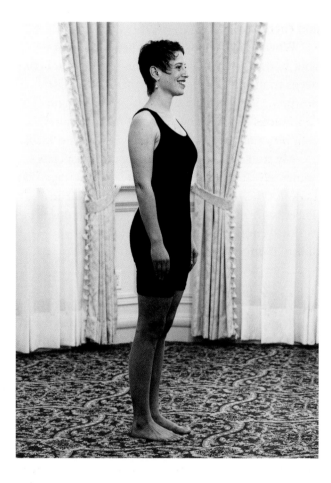

PROPER STANDING ALIGNMENT

Health is wealth. Peace of mind is happiness.
Yoga shows the way.

— SWAMI VISHNU-DEVANANDA

Throughout the twelve main chapters, you will see the instructions "Come into Proper Standing Alignment." Before you practice any posture, it is necessary to align your body so that the yoga posture is not only safe, but also effective and beneficial. Practice this standing posture whenever you can: as you wait in line, talk to friends, make dinner. Even when you are lying on your belly, you can elongate the body using an adapted version of this process. I teach my students to memorize key parts of the body, from the feet up to the crown of the head.

Let's begin:

1. **Feet**. Yoga is practiced in bare feet. First, the feet are placed directly under the hips. They are parallel. Imagine that each foot is a car with four wheels at the bottom. Evenly distribute your weight on these four wheels, so that most of the foot is in contact with the floor. Spread the toes for balance.

2. **Thighs**. Engage the thighs by actively lifting them away from the knees.

3. **Pelvic Floor**. This area of the body, the pubococcygeal (or PC) muscles, may be difficult to isolate at first. One way is to imagine that you are attempting to stop the flow of urine. (Women know this inner lift as Kegel exercises, commonly recommended by doctors to strengthen bladder control and to help prevent damage to the birth canal during delivery. For our purposes here, however, the same principles apply to both men and women.) When activated in this way, the PC muscles form a foundation of internal support during the postures. You'll notice that your buttocks tighten automatically during the inner lift. This is essential as a means to protect the back, particularly during back-bending postures. Be sure to breathe while you squeeze these muscles. (The inner lift is an advanced technique, so don't be discouraged if you can't do it right away. It will become easier after you have developed your knowledge of the postures.)

4. **Tailbone/Buttocks**. Tuck in the tailbone *slightly*. Do not overdo this movement by pressing the pelvis forward. Your lower back has a natural curve that should be maintained.

5. **Waist**. For a moment, place your hands on your hips and imagine that you are trying to lift your torso up out of your waist. Wiggle up and side-to-side to accentuate this idea. Relax your arms back down to your sides.

6. **Chest**. Imagine two points on either side of your

chest between your nipples and your collar bone. Pretend that they have marionette strings attached to them and that someone is lifting you up toward the ceiling. This is not the same as the military stance where you throw your chest out in front of you. Rather, it lengthens the spine and keeps the torso long and tall.

7. **Shoulders**. Many of us carry so much tension in our shoulders that it has become habitual. To understand the relationship between where your shoulders sit when they are relaxed and when they are tense, use the technique of exaggeration. Inhale and lift the shoulders up around your ears as if you were trying to hide your neck. Exhale forcefully and drop the shoulders. This is where they need to be for Proper Standing Alignment. Repeat several times to let go of any tension that may be stored in your shoulders.

8. **Crown of the Head**. Imagine again that you are a marionette. The main string that helps you to stand upright is located at the crown of the head. Press the top of your head up as if you were trying to touch it to the ceiling. Be sure not to jut the head or chin forward or upward. If you have a tendency to do this, simply tuck the chin slightly and draw the head back over the spine.

9. **Corners of the Mouth.** When you turn up the corners of your mouth, you are forming an attitudinal posture, called smiling. It's amazing what happens to us when we choose to smile. Go ahead and try it!

10. **Breathe!** At first, this series of points to remember may feel unnatural and awkward. The more you practice them, the easier they will become. Within a week or two, Proper Standing Alignment will feel like second nature, and you will *want* to stand in this manner. Maintain an even, steady breathing pattern so that you feel comfortable in this significant stance.

ABOUT CREATING YOUR OWN POSTURE

This may strike you as unusual in a yoga book. You might say, "Hey, I picked up this book to learn the formal yoga postures, not to have to figure them out on my own." The traditional postures described in this book may be five thousand years old, but they were still created with peoples' bodies just like yours or mine. When you put on your favorite music in your living room and start to dance around, you are not concerned with whether or not your ballet instructor would approve of your footing. Your body has innate wisdom and knows how to move in ways that make it feel good, strong, and energized.

When you create your own posture, listen to your body. Notice which way your energy wants or needs to move. You may come up with a single posture, a series of poses, or a spontaneous and continuous flow of movement. If music inspires you, play some that will enhance your inward focus.

My students enjoy this part of our yoga class immensely. It becomes even clearer at this stage that I am not the teacher; rather, we are all teachers. There is great power in creating your own postures: they will connect you most intimately to your Spiritual Muscles.

ABOUT THE BREATHING LESSONS

Without proper breathing, the yoga postures are nothing more than mere calisthenics. You can have a beautiful chandelier with gorgeous dangling crystals, but without electricity, they will never flash and sparkle. Your breath is the energy that supports the postures. Some of the breathing lessons will seem strange to you. Give them the time and space you would a flower to blossom. The results these techniques can yield will amaze you.

I often tell my students that if they learn no other skill to carry with them throughout their lives, at least learn how to *breathe* properly. Often, they look at me in puzzlement with eyes that say, "But we already *are* breathing, aren't we?" Well, of course we are all breathing to some extent. But most of us are not breathing fully, nor are we using our maximum lung capacity.

As babies, most of us took full, deep, and natural breaths. Have you ever noticed an infant breathing when she sleeps? Her belly goes OUT and IN, OUT and IN rhythmically. She is not lying there wondering what her belly looks like, trying to pull in her gut, or worried about what size jeans she wears.

If we all started off this way, what happened that led most of us astray? The answer is—a lot! Daily stressors and tensions imprison our breathing apparatus. Our emotions are also mirrored in our breath. You can tell how you are feeling by noticing how you are breathing. Because our emotional life is so closely linked to our breath, we can look to our breath for guidance and clarity when we are unclear about our feelings.

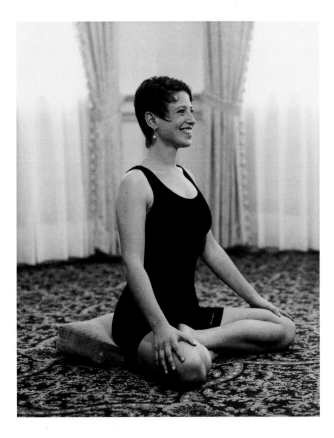

PROPER SITTING ALIGNMENT

For most of the Breathing Lessons (with the exception of the Sun Breath, The Breath of Joy, and Abdominal Contractions), you will be in a comfortable seated position. It's easy to fall into the habit of sitting in what I call "TV mode": back hunched over, shoulders rounded forward, and no spinal support. Your head reaches forward as if the volume is too low and you are straining to hear. To overcome this unhealthy seated posture, follow the following instructions for Proper Sitting Alignment. It is helpful to sit on a meditation cushion or a rolled-up towel. Meditation benches are great too, since they keep your hips raised above your knees,

and the seat is angled to support Proper Sitting Alignment. As a beginner, you will find it easiest to sit cross-legged on the floor (shown) or in a chair. You may need to place a pillow or a rolled-up towel under one or both knees for support.

Let's begin:

1. **Sitting Bones**. These are the two knobs at the base of your pelvis. Take a moment to walk back and forth from one side of the buttocks to the other, until you find them. Instead of plopping down in the middle of your cushion or rolled-up towel, sit on the edge of the cushion directly atop these bones. This will help to align your spinal column and enable you to maintain the natural curve of your lower spine without exaggerating it.

2. **Waist**. Place your hands on your hips and imagine that you are lifting your torso up out of your waist. Wiggle up and side-to-side. Make sure that your abdomen is not compressed. Your spine is long. Now, rest your hands either comfortably on your knees or in your lap.

3. **Chest**. Imagine two points on either side of your chest between your nipples and your collar bone. Pretend that they have marionette strings attached to them and that someone is lifting them up toward the ceiling.

4. **Shoulders**. Inhale and lift the shoulders up around your ears as if you are trying to hide your neck. Exhale forcefully and drop the shoulders. This is where they need to be for Proper Sitting Alignment. Repeat several times to let go of any tension that may be stored in your shoulders.

5. **Crown of the Head**. Imagine again that you are a marionette. The main string that keeps you upright is located at the crown of the head. Press the top of your head up as if you are trying to touch it to the ceiling. Be sure not to jut the head or chin forward or upward. If you have a tendency to do this, simply tuck in the chin slightly and draw the head back over the spine.

ABOUT THE RELAXATIONS/ VISUALIZATIONS/MEDITATIONS

Relaxing involves the whole person. There is no point in having a relaxed body if your mind still races at sixty miles per hour. Similarly, it is of little use to have a calm, peaceful mind if the body is tense and tight. Body and mind affect each other. When one is calm and centered, the other can follow more easily.

Have a trustworthy person read the relaxation to you, or read it into a tape recorder yourself. Have paper, magic markers, crayons, or pens nearby, as you may wish to write or draw at the end of the experience. Be sure that you will be undisturbed, that the lights are low, and that you have a sweater or a blanket nearby in case you get cool.

The concept of "doing nothing" is foreign to most of us. If we do nothing, we believe we are either lazy, unmotivated, or sick. I encourage my students to take five-minute breaks throughout the day to relax and do nothing—without guilt. Those mere five minutes can act as a thermostat and help to balance and regulate your energy. You will return to your day refreshed, enthusiastic, productive, efficient, and content.

The truth is that both relaxation and visualization (the process of imagining an event or scene in the mind with as much clarity, feeling, and detail as possible) require conscious effort. And like cooking or tennis, they are skills that improve with practice. Unfortunately, most people visualize through disempowering and energy-depleting mental habits like worrying. Consider a cold, wintry morning. What pictures flood your mind when you hear a storm forecast on the radio? Do you see car accidents and traffic jams? Do you already feel nervous even though you are still in bed under the covers? This kind of imaging is self-defeating. Put yourself in the driver's seat of your visualization experiences by seeing the traffic flowing smoothly and safely. You can be outrageously creative and have fun in the process!

Some days, you'll decide that you have time only for the postures and breathing techniques, and will want to skip the relaxation. *Resist that urge.* Ending a yoga session without a relaxation is like going to a birthday party and skipping the cake.

THE CORPSE POSE

At the end of your yoga session, you will come into your favorite variation of the Corpse Pose, the posture of relaxation. This is ideal for guided visualizations. It is in the Corpse Pose that you can truly integrate the benefits of yoga. You may choose to come into the Corpse Pose between each posture as a way to renew yourself before beginning the next one.

Do not skip this posture. Take time for relaxation after every yoga session. It may seem simple, yet for many people, it is the most difficult pose of all. The Corpse Pose emphasizes simply *being*, while our culture is focused on *doing*.

In the beginning, you may find that you drift in and out of awareness, but try to stay awake in the Corpse Pose. You already know how to relax when you are unconscious (that's called "sleeping"). The challenge and benefits of the Corpse Pose come from relaxing while you are conscious.

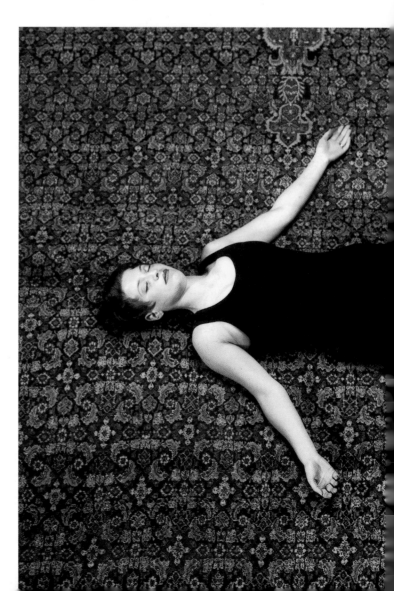

When to avoid this posture If you are in the sixth month of pregnancy or beyond, avoid lying on your back for long periods of time, as this puts pressure on the vena cava, the large blood vessel that runs in back of the uterus. Instead, lie on your left side with your knees bent and use pillows between the knees and anywhere else that enhances your comfort.

Let's begin:

1. Come into a position lying on your back with your legs extended out on the floor. Allow your eyes to close gently. **Variation**: If you have any lower back discomfort, bend the knees farther than hip width apart and place your feet on the floor. Rest the knees against each other and focus on keeping your lower back pressed into the floor.

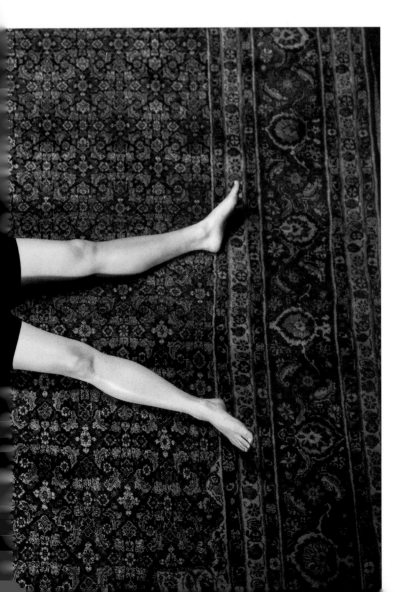

2. Rest your arms a few inches from your sides, palms up in a position of receptivity.

3. Separate your feet about hip width apart. As you relax the feet they naturally turn out in opposite directions.

4. Be sure that your spine is long and that your body is symmetrical. For example, each arm should be the same distance from your body and at a similar angle.

5. Adjust your position with micromovements that enhance your comfort.

6. Be aware of tensions in your body. You don't need to use any muscle in this posture. Scan the body for tensions: the face, eyes, jaw, belly, hands, et cetera. Invite all of these areas to let go and consciously direct your breath to them.

7. Focus on your breath. Feel your breath coming in and going out of the body.

8. When you are ready to come out of the Corpse Pose, move slowly. It is as though you just woke up from a restful nap. Begin by deepening your breath and feeling your body in contact with the floor beneath you. Wiggle your fingertips and toes before moving any other part of the body.

9. Finally, curl over onto one side, resting for a moment in the fetal position. Transition gradually by bringing your body back into a comfortable seated position.

WHAT YOGA IS AND ISN'T

I went from thinking yoga was just sitting with your legs crossed and humming to having a whole world open up before me.

—AMALIA ACEVEDO-MIRASOLA,
YOGA STUDENT

On the first day of class, I ask my students to find a partner and tell each other everything they have heard about yoga, even if it seems weird or unusual. After the students have had a chance to compare notes, I tally the results. I inevitably hear at least the following four ideas:

➤ Yoga is some kind of yogurt.

➤ Yoga is a cult.

➤ Yoga is an old man with his legs crossed chanting "OOOHMMM."

➤ Yoga is twisting the body into a pretzel.

Of course, I also hear other more accurate answers. I'd like to comment on the four above first, just to alleviate any residual or nagging thoughts in the back of your mind.

➤ **Yoga is NOT some kind of yogurt.** The biggest similarity between yoga and yogurt is that the first three letters are the same. Actually, the word *yoga* is a Sanskrit term meaning "union." The only other words in the American Heritage Dictionary that start with these three letters are *yogh*, a letter of the Middle English alphabet; *Yogyakarta*, a city in Java; and *yogi*, a person who practices yoga—hey, that's you!

➤ **Yoga is NOT a cult.** To me, a cult is a scary group of people who try to take you away from what you know and who you are. Yoga is the opposite. It reminds you that everything you need to know is inside of you and brings you closer to who you are. It is a system of combining physical stretches with deep breathing and relaxation that invites you to open up to all of your possibilities.

➤ **Yoga is NOT an old man with his legs crossed chanting "OOOHMMM."** Actually, there are many old men doing yoga, and not just the yogis and masters living in India. However, all types of people of any age, race, gender, or religion can and do practice yoga. And while many yoga practitioners have discovered a great benefit from chanting certain sounds such as *om*, chanting is not a requirement. Many yoga classes do begin and end by chanting *om* in order to relax and unify the group.

➤ **Yoga is NOT twisting the body into a pretzel.** Part of yoga involves Flexibility, both of body and, more importantly, of mind. Yoga is a five-thousand-year-old science of self-improvement. One type of yoga, which I call the Royal Yoga of Body and Mind, focuses on moving the physical body into certain positions or *postures*. These postures stimulate the musculoskeletal system and all internal organs and systems to work more effectively and efficiently. Some of these postures may seem strange the first time you do them, especially if you are accustomed to the habitual postures of standing, sitting, and lying down. With practice the postures will become easier. Believe it or not, we have already achieved one of the most difficult positions: according to one developmental psychology text, learning to stand and walk on our own is one of the most difficult challenges that we face in our lifetime. Congratulations—you have already accomplished a great feat!

WHAT ARE THE BENEFITS OF YOGA?

I think of yoga as a lifetime ticket on American Airlines. Yoga is going to take me wherever I need to go. It has the capability of increasing confidence, interpersonal skills, happiness, peace, love, success, and all the dreams that life is made up of.

—MARJORIE GANDOLFO,
YOGA STUDENT

Although there are numerous spiritual qualities you can develop with yoga, some of the benefits fall under the umbrella of the twelve Spiritual Muscles: Awareness, Acceptance, Focus, Flexibility, Balance, Confidence, Peace, Strength, Compassion, Energy, Playfulness, and Connectedness. Focusing on one of the Spiritual Muscles at a time is both helpful and practical. Benjamin Franklin, aside from his publishing and political work, was a master at the art of self-improvement and concentration. He chose one quality per week to develop in himself and focused on it. This book encourages you to do just that.

However, there are more tangible benefits that occur when people practice yoga on a regular basis. I've experienced them myself and have seen them in my students. According to their journals, my students sleep better, concentrate more easily on their jobs and studies, feel more self-assured, relate to others more effectively, manage stress and distress, improve their sex lives, lose weight in a health-oriented manner, and change habits to improve their all-around state of well-being. Here are some specific examples:

➤ At least one or two students in every class each semester announce that they have eliminated or reduced episodes of panic attacks.

➤ One woman shared with the class that she lost thirty-three pounds in one semester.

➤ An older student proclaimed that she no longer needs blood-pressure medication, since she began daily yoga and relaxation.

➤ One student broke an eight-year, two-pack-a-day cigarette habit with deep abdominal breathing (essentially the same inhalation and exhalation process as taking a drag on a cigarette).

➤ Another student credits yoga for improving his sexual relationship with his partner.

Students of yoga are more confident speaking in front of groups and generally have a positive, pro-active attitude. Many find that yoga improves their athletic and musical performance. In fact whatever you do, you'll do it better once yoga is a regular part of your life.

Some students have gained new insights and developed coping skills for eating disorders, drug use, low-grade depression, inability to concentrate, and managing emotions (particularly anger). They have built a foundation of self-esteem, self-trust, and self-responsibility that will last a lifetime. They pass along these benefits to others through teaching and role modeling.

Because yoga is about developing Awareness and tuning into the body, students are better able to listen to their bodies' messages. For example, yoga in and of itself did not strip my student of thirty-three pounds; yoga offered her the opportunity to attune to her body and her spirit's true needs. Instead of allowing her fears to take the lead, she learned self-confidence and how to trust the wisdom of her body.

When we really listen to the body, we may get messages we don't always like. Many of my students say that when they first begin yoga, they become aware of how out of shape they are, how tired they are, how nervous and unrelaxed they are. This is a good sign. Increased awareness enables you to begin to take better care of the incredible vehicle that has been serving you all these years.

A final note: you may get benefits from yoga you didn't expect. I invite you to remain open to the possibilities that are inherent in loving and caring for your body.

HOW CAN I FIND TIME FOR YOGA?

Allowing myself the time for yoga really relieves any tension or stress. It's like unwinding a tight ball of yarn.

—JAIMIE ADKINS, YOGA STUDENT

I wake up early and before I do anything else, I walk into my yoga room and begin my practice to physically, mentally, emotionally, and spiritually prepare myself for the day. Afterward, I feel more awake and refreshed, and I have more emotional balance and psychological vigor. Any time of the day, however (except right after a meal), is a good time to do yoga. Find the time that works best for you.

Of the twenty-four hours in each day, how many do you spend taking care of your body—moving, breathing deeply, stretching, and relaxing? Many people say they just don't have time to take care of their bodies. But if you don't have time for your body, eventually your body won't have time for you!

Each chapter in *Yoga for Your Spiritual Muscles* contains a complete yoga session. To find the time, you may have to get up a little earlier or spend less time in the shower. Or you may have to turn the TV off sooner at night. Giving yourself the gift of yoga will help you to sleep better and wake up more refreshed.

OVERCOMING EXCUSES

Before I started yoga class, I was so lazy. I hit the snooze button on my clock at least four times before I got myself out of bed.

—TAMARA SZWECKI, YOGA STUDENT

— I'm too busy.

— I'm too tired.

— I'm too fat.

— This is too difficult.

9

— I'm lazy.

— I might hurt myself.

— This is weird.

— I'm not flexible enough.

— My dog ate this book.

We all come up with reasons for not wanting to do yoga and other healthy activities because the pain seems to outweigh the pleasure. It really does boil down to just that: pain versus pleasure. We would all like the pleasure of having done an hour of yoga and relaxation, but sometimes we decide to take a nap, watch TV, sleep, or eat instead. Taken to an extreme, this is known as *resistance*. Recognizing our resistance is the first step before we can take action to move beyond it.

When you do come up with reasons why you can't possibly do yoga, try instead to be your own mental cheerleader. What are all of the pleasures, benefits, and good feelings you'll get if you practice yoga? Inspire yourself by focusing on what you'll gain by doing even ten minutes of yoga. For example, in the short run you'll gain renewed energy and vitality, while over the long term you'll improve your confidence and strengthen your immune system.

If that isn't enough, you can also motivate yourself with the consequences of *not* doing yoga. What are all of the things you'll lose by not doing yoga today, tomorrow, for the next few months, two years, or more? You may say "I'll lose my flexibility, my self-esteem, my connection to my body, my temper, my concentration." Use the energy of these negatives to align yourself with that positive and encouraging expression, "Just do it."

Keep in mind that the stages of a spiritual relationship are identical to the stages of any intimate relationship. The honeymoon phase in our marriage to spirit is often filled with overwhelming joy and a satisfying sense of wholeness. Like any worthwhile relationship, a spiritual one has its share of doubt, loneliness, anger, and any other experience you may have with a special partner. Your vow to maintain your dedication to wholeness is "for richer or poorer." Allow your connection with spirit the space to encounter the richness of a full and meaningful path.

TEN STEPS TO CREATING AN AMBIANCE FOR YOGA

I've been practicing yoga in my dorm room since the semester started, and I notice that the room feels different to me now. It feels more like a sanctuary than a cell.

—JACK LUTRIS, YOGA STUDENT

To have a sacred place . . . is an absolute necessity for anybody today. You must have a room, or a certain hour or so a day, where . . . you can simply experience and bring forth what you are and what you might be. This is a place of creative incubation. At first you may find that nothing happens there. But if you have a sacred place and use it, something eventually will happen.

—JOSEPH CAMPBELL, *THE POWER OF MYTH*

The size of your yoga space does not need to be large. You will need a space on the floor that is long enough to comfortably lie down on with room enough to reach your hands over your head and out to the sides. Here are some ideas:

1. Review the room or area in your home with the least amount of traffic. For example, if you live in a two-story space with the main entrance on the first floor, find a spot upstairs. Put a sign on your door, if necessary, that reads "Quiet Please: Becoming Enlightened" or something similar. If your location is noisy beyond your control, use the sounds to draw you deeper within yourself by allowing them to become a part of your yoga experience. Remind yourself that, although the world around you may be loud and chaotic, your inner experience can be quiet and calm.

2. Bring a few favorite objects into the space. You may have photographs of loved ones, role models, or beautiful, inspiring places. Surround yourself with stones, shells, flowers, or anything that reminds you of your spirit. Let your imagination run wild.

3. Keep the space clean and uncluttered. Often our external space mirrors our internal experience and vice-versa. If your surroundings are neat and

comfortable, you will tend to have a similar internal feeling. Create an aesthetically pleasing place that will be a joy for you to practice in.

4. Listen to inspiring music. Or open the windows to the sound of birds, the rain, or even the traffic. Avoid catchy music that draws you out of an internal focus.

5. Explore different means of enhancing your space through smell by investigating aromatherapy, incense, or scented candles. Your olfactory sense is more significant to your experience than you might think. Would you rather smell lavender or a pile of dirty socks?

6. Eliminate harsh, direct, and overhead lighting. Replace it with soft, indirect lighting. Try candles occasionally for a special effect. Be sure the candles are out of the way of your physical movement— just in case.

7. Make your space as physically comfortable as possible. Use a room with a rug or get a sturdy mat. Keep soft pillows available, both for props and for comfort.

8. If possible, do not eat where you practice yoga. But do keep a glass of water nearby. Never allow yourself become dehydrated.

9. Make sure you have good airflow and that your space gets fresh air as often as possible. Breathing full, deep breaths requires clean air in order to be effective and nourishing. Keep the space free from polluted or stale air.

10. When you are away from home, consider what space you will use so that your routine remains steadfast and uninterrupted.

TEN RULES FOR BUILDING SPIRITUAL MUSCLES

I learned a lot about my body, and how to exercise more than just my muscles.

—BRIAN SEGEDIN, YOGA STUDENT

1. **Know Your Limits.** If you have any pre-existing medical conditions, please consult your doctor before beginning any exercise program. Always stop if you feel pain or discomfort. Move in and out of postures *slowly.* Pay attention to the limitations noted for each posture. Modify postures to suit your body's needs. Never force yourself, physically or otherwise. For example, if you are mourning a loss, postures that encourage an open heart may not be in your best interest, especially right away. Remember, you know your body better than anyone.

2. **Listen to Your Body.** Sometimes there is a fine line between the messages of your body and your mind. Your mind is very talkative and may object to certain postures. "Hey! I'm not sure I want to be in this position. Forget this yoga thing!" In reality, your body may be very capable of doing the posture even though your mind is trying to talk you out of it. Practice listening to your body and it will reward you with great benefits.

3. **Breathe.** The words *spirit* and *inspire* have the same root, which means "to breathe." Try to breathe as fully as possible before, during, and after each posture.

4. **Expand Your Comfort Zone.** Go beyond what you think you can do. Do not continue if you feel any sharp pain, but be aware that minor discomforts come with the territory and are normal. Most of us live in a little box called "my comfort zone" that limits how we act, look, feel, and express ourselves. By expanding our comfort zone, we explore our possibilities. Start small and build on your successes. Your definition of who you are will also expand. The sky's the limit!

5. **Have Fun!** Watch children play and let them be your role models. Don't take yoga so seriously that you forget to enjoy it.

6. **Let Go of Self-Judgment.** Be aware of self-judgment during your yoga practice. Voices of fear or disappointment might visit you. "Gee, I still can't touch my toes after practicing the Flexibility chapter. I'm always so stiff and achy. I feel like I'm twenty years older than my true age." Be gentle and patient with yourself as you would when a child is first learning how to walk. Let yourself be a beginner. And even after you become comfortable with the postures, maintain an attitude of freshness, awe, and wonder toward this miracle that is your body.

7. **Be Comfortable.** Wear loose, flexible clothing that you feel good wearing and moving in. Avoid clothes that constrict your breathing during yoga and in your daily life.

8. **Eat Lightly.** Try to eat no less than two hours prior to your yoga practice. This makes early morning or before meals ideal times. Eating moderately will enable you to feel light and more energetic.

9. **Make This *Your* Time.** Tell yourself that for a specific period of time, you will put aside your worries, fears, troubles, and responsibilities. This is your time to focus on the essence of who you are. Make sure the phone is off the hook or the answering machine is on. Let family and friends know that you will be unavailable. This is not selfish. Rather, by giving ourselves time to grow and develop, we are more able to give to others.

10. **Create a Routine for Yourself.** Practicing at the same time each day is very helpful. The more you practice yoga, the more you will see and feel the benefits. On days when you do not practice, you will notice the difference in your mood, your flexibility, and your temperament. Practicing yoga is not only vital, it also prepares you for the day ahead—it loosens the body, calms the mind, balances the emotions, and focuses your energy. By maintaining consistency, you create a spiritual ritual that will nourish your inner and outer being.

THE MANY BRANCHES OF YOGA

Like a bountiful fruit tree, yoga contains many branches, all with the same aim: union. This book encourages you to practice all of yoga's branches: the Yoga of Service (Karma Yoga), the Yoga of Devotion (Bhakti Yoga), the Yoga of Knowledge (Jnana Yoga), and the Royal Yoga of Body and Mind (Hatha and Raja Yoga).

Just as you choose a major to study in college, most people choose to focus on one path of yoga. But in the University of Life you can practice all of the paths, which will deepen your relationship to spirit and help you to achieve union that much more effectively.

Did you ever leave a gift at someone's door, ring the doorbell, and then run away? You were practicing the Yoga of Service. The Yoga of Service enables you to be lovingly transformed through your work or your duties while letting go of the fruits of your labor. The Yoga of Service has less to do with *what* you do, than with *how* you do it. Mother Teresa was a beautiful example of the Yoga of Service, of someone who devoted her life to helping others unselfishly. As you practice the Royal Yoga of Body and Mind and connect more intimately with yourself, you will naturally want to share yoga with others.

Can you recall a time when you read a deeply moving poem, heard an inspirational song, or watched a breathtaking sunset and felt a profound sense of oneness with the universe? At that moment you experienced the Yoga of Devotion. When we allow ourselves to achieve this kind of mystical merging, we surrender to seeing the highest in everything. This intense path enables emotional passion and heartfelt feeling to guide the way to the sacred.

The Yoga of Knowledge doesn't involve book learning as much as direct knowledge through experience. It's the difference between watching a travelogue and living with a native family in a foreign country. Your deepest understanding will come from *doing* yoga, from understanding your inner and outer experiences during practice.

The Royal Yoga of Body and Mind is the main path of this book. But saying that you take a yoga class is like saying that you take a dance class. What kind is it? Ballet, jazz, Afro-Cuban, musical theater, and West Coast swing are just a few of the myriad dance forms. Yet they differ tremendously—as do the various schools in this branch of yoga.

All schools of yoga teach basically the same postures. Some are more vigorous, others more gentle. Some branches teach the postures in a flow, others foster a more static approach. Certain schools emphasize precision with eyes open, while others offer basic alignment with eyes closed to find your own inner movement. Some require your room to be 110 degrees Fahrenheit, others practice yoga outdoors.

This book teaches a delightful middle path. It can be as vigorous or gentle as you make it. You can create a flow of the postures or take minibreaks after each posture to integrate its benefits. *Yoga for Your*

Spiritual Muscles offers structural alignment without getting caught up in too much detail. Listen to the wisdom of your body. You can keep your eyes open or closed as your mood moves you. Though I recommend a warm room for your practice, I encourage you to practice in a space that feels appropriate and comfortable to you.

As you practice the Royal Yoga of Body and Mind, consider yourself a King or Queen of yoga! Remember, the external postures are the path to the internal postures.

All of the paths of yoga complement each other in their aims and come together to form a balanced whole. These four major schools of yoga have similar qualities to the four elements honored by many cultures. The Yoga of Devotion represents the heart or *water* element and highlights the relationships and emotional connections in our lives. The Yoga of Knowledge signifies the *air* element that addresses the intellectual and mental functions. Like *fire*, the Yoga of Service symbolizes action. Finally, the Royal Yoga of Body and Mind connects us to the *earth* in the here and now, grounding our spirits in the moment.

THERE'S NOTHING BETTER THAN A GREAT TEACHER

Regardless of the particular path of yoga, you will find it helpful to have a teacher. A good teacher is one with whom you resonate and who serves as a spiritual guide. Throughout your life, you may be lucky enough to have many teachers. Initially you may find a teacher to inspire and encourage you to practice safely and correctly. Later, you may find someone to both challenge and assure you. Show this book to your teacher and your class. Sharing your growth and excitement inspires others. There are many ways to cross the threshold into the world of spirit. Let your passages be filled with support, trust, and camaraderie.

THE ART OF KEEPING A YOGA JOURNAL

The practice of yoga is complemented by thoughtful journal keeping. Your experiences are worth recording. Through journaling, you can see how much you have changed, grown, and learned.

Something happens to us when we journal. If we are afraid, our fears dissipate. When we are confused, we become clearer. When we are sad, we feel like we've shared some of the burden with a nonjudgmental friend. At the same time, our joys and successes become more real and valid when we write them down. It's like an inexpensive form of therapy.

The journal does not have to read like a chronological autobiography. In fact, that's part of the beauty of journal writing. It can contain a quote here, a story there, a drawing of a visualization, a special list. Feel free to add photographs, collages, poems, or anything else that feels relevant or significant to you.

Free yourself from the "perfect journal" concept—it's a trap. Let your yoga journal become an expression of who you are at different moments. You can record how you felt before, during, or after practicing yoga. Mark significant ways that yoga affects other areas of your life. If possible, try to capture thoughts and feelings as quickly as you can after they have happened. Memories, like dreams, tend to fade as time elapses.

Journaling can provide valuable insights. Often when things are tumbling around in your head, it is difficult to gain clarity on an issue. When you write it all down, it is as if all of the great masters and teachers that live inside you have a chance to be heard. Reading over your journal—days, months, or even years later—you may be astonished to recognize that the glimmerings of major changes in your life were mirrored in your thoughts and dreams long before they became conscious. Thus, you can develop a greater Awareness of your own patterns of development and growth.

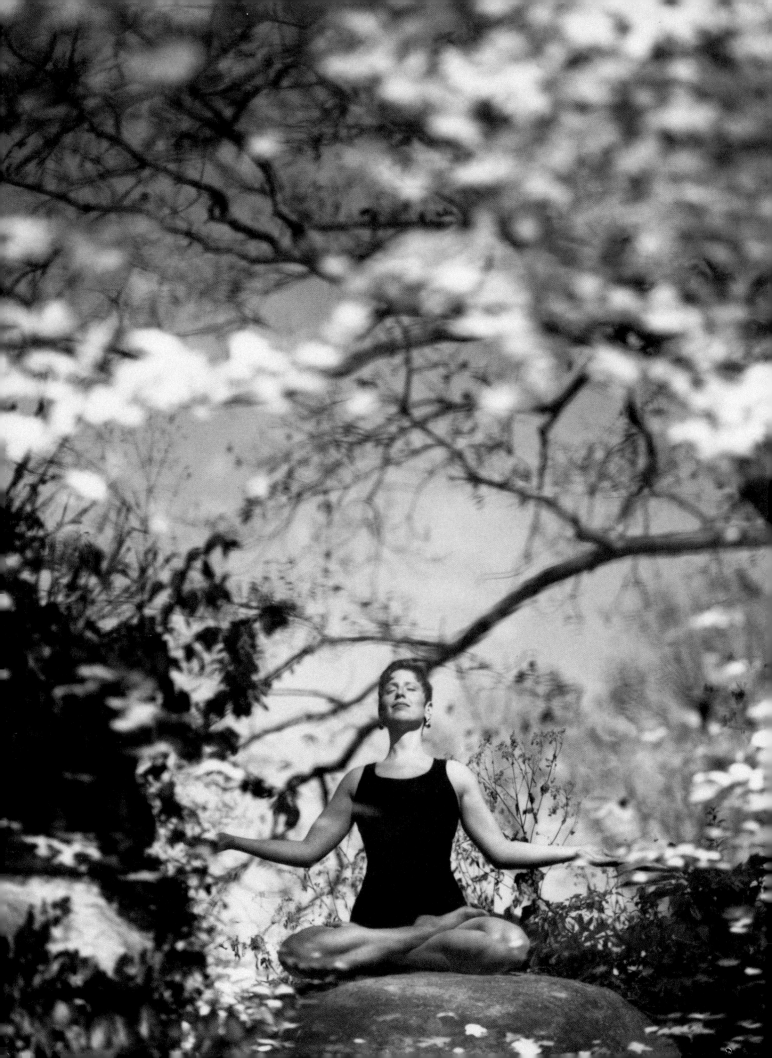

AWARENESS

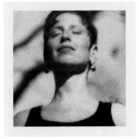

One of my colleagues has a watch with no hour or second hand. It has on it only the word NOW. Life's greatest gifts are available when we are in the present moment. In worrying about the future or lamenting the past, the present gets lost. When we open ourselves to the present moment, all we need to do is to be.

If we want to make changes or improvements in our lives, we must first become conscious of what is actually going on now. Learning to pay attention is the foundation for the development of a relationship with ourselves. Only when we are mindful of the present moment can we truly embrace the richness of life and make room for all of the experiences it has to offer.

Children can teach us the art of "beginner's mind." They see the world through fresh, open eyes. To begin to develop the Spiritual Muscle of Awareness, try looking at a flower as if for the very first time. See all of the amazing tones of color. What feelings does this flower evoke in you? Feel the nuances of texture in the petals, the leaves, and the stem. Inhale its unique scent. Consider what it would feel like to *be* a flower. If it's a rose or a marigold, taste it as though you are an epicure of divine food. Flowers and other parts of nature are not burdened by confusion about who and what they are.

Awareness for us humans is partly a matter of waking up to the truth that we already are the miracle we wish to be. This awakening comes first from letting go of all that thwarts us from that inherent truth. Being present is as much a matter of going deeper as it is of widening and expanding our consciousness. When our consciousness is clear and open, it's as though a veil screening our eyes from the real view has been lifted.

Our breath is the gateway for developing Awareness. From our first breath at birth to our last at death, breath is a constant companion and a mirror for our feelings. How do you breathe when you are nervous or afraid? Choppy and shallow? When you are relaxed the breath is smooth, deep, and full. Take your emotional and mental temperature by tuning into your ever-present inhalation and exhalation. Each breath is unique and encapsulates your current state of being.

Cultivating Awareness through meditation on the breath or in some other form is at the heart of most ancient traditions. In modern times, meditation is making a comeback as an antidote to the disease of our culture, stress. But it is not that easy to be truly mindful. All meditation systems describe the same difficulties and disturbances of mind and heart.

I take step aerobic classes and I just do whatever the teacher does. I never really think about how my body feels and whether or not I can do what she's doing. I just follow along. It had never occurred to me that I should be listening to what is happening internally. Since I've started yoga, I try to feel my body benefiting from what I'm doing, while I do it. It's a whole new way of caring for my body.

— MEG OTTO-MCLEAR, YOGA STUDENT

During meditation, we begin to notice the texture of these hindrances. Gradually we become less tangled up in our negative emotions such as anger, fear, hate, our unending desires, laziness, restlessness, and doubt. As Awareness grows, our behavior shifts, and inner transformation begins.

When you are in a helping capacity, meditation can also foster healing in others. As author and meditation teacher Stephen Levine says in *Healers on Healing*:

> *One can become so sensitive in deeper levels of meditation practice that one's body can become like a fine-tuned diagnostic instrument. Then by feeling various changes in one's body and mind while with a client, one can understand something deeper of the client's inner experience and illness. Many techniques and therapies are useful, but nothing is as effective as daily meditation practice to deepen the well from which the thirst for healing may be slaked. Meditation develops the sensitivity needed to use any method of healing with skill and effectiveness.*

Yoga is the moving meditation that teaches us Awareness through bodily sensations that arise during the postures. Become absorbed in the rich subtleties of each movement. While you hold or move through each yoga posture, allow all of your Awareness to remain internal. Become a nonjudgmental observer, uncovering facts without forming an opinion. Unlike a court of law that judges innocence or guilt, in yoga we simply witness all of the body's sensations.

See if you can go beyond the habitual verdicts such as pain (it's uncomfortable) or pleasure (it feels good). Unless the feeling is distinctly sharp pain (in which case *stop immediately!*), go to the heart of the sensations and explore them. Notice what is happening in the moment without trying to make it other than what it is. As we use witness consciousness to effect change, we discover the first steps to inner growth.

Postures for Awareness Experiment with closing the eyes in the Six Movements of the Spine, Runner's Stretch, Five-Pointed Star, and Half-Moon. Awareness deepens when your eyes are closed and you tune out extraneous stimuli. The Face Massage is a delightful way to become conscious of relaxing the muscles of the face.

Breathing Lesson for Awareness The Natural Breath is the most basic yogic breathing technique. Let it become a rewarding foundation for developing your Awareness.

Relaxation for Awareness Private "I" Investigation is a thorough experience of scanning the body for both discomfort and joy.

My older sister is very sick with Hodgkin's disease. She is twenty-five and has always been my idol and, in a way, my mentor. I admire her now more than ever as she battles her illness. I used to say "Why us?" but now I'm glad she has a chance to survive rather than dying suddenly, as in a car accident. I no longer feel that she is slowly dying. Instead, I feel she is slowly recovering. I have never been such a positive person, and the only thing I can attribute this to is yoga.

— PATTY NELSON, YOGA STUDENT

YOGA STORY FOR AWARENESS:
JEFF MIGDOW, M.D. (PRABHAKAR)

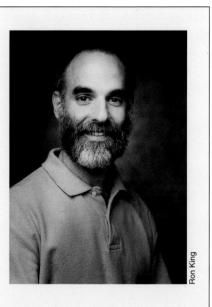

Ron King

Jeff Migdow is a holistic doctor with a practice in Lenox, Massachusetts. He encourages his patients to learn how to breathe, relax, and do yoga—all to develop their Awareness. In some cases, he's helped folks avoid surgery. He is a person who sincerely walks his talk.

Originally during my yoga practice, I became aware of how *unaware* I was. I would keep coming back to the sensations and try to bring my mind back to myself when it wandered. Then I started to notice where my mind went, and I could catch it and bring it back. I was more present—which allowed me to be more energetic and focused.

My yoga experience and my medical practice changed. My whole life revolved around being aware of whether or not I was present. When I could bring myself back to the present moment, my life became much easier, smoother, and joyous. I could reach the goals that I set while feeling more relaxed. When I wasn't able to do this, I became more tense. It was more challenging for me to feel energetic and fulfilled and more difficult to get things done.

Most people have problem areas in their lives that would benefit from change. I encourage my patients to become aware of the situations in their lives that may be causing their symptoms—and what experiences help them heal: what foods, activities, and what people affect them.

One patient came to me after another doctor suggested surgery for severe shoulder and upper back pain. He had osteoporosis and arthritis in his cervical spine, and his vertebrae were compressed. I taught him simple yoga stretches and encouraged him to do them with Awareness. My instructions were "If you feel pain, pull back." When I saw him ten days later, he had experienced periods of relief. Two weeks later, he improved further with still less pain. Continuing his simple but effective yoga practice, within a few months he decided to put the surgery off altogether.

When people do yoga consistently they're much more open to change. That's the key: If I'm not open to making changes, then I won't let myself be aware. What's the point of being aware if I'm not going to listen to my Awareness and act on it?

It is only through a change in human consciousness that the world will be transformed. The personal and the planetary are connected. As we expand our awareness of body, mind, psyche, and spirit, so also will the world be changed. This is our quest as we explore New Dimensions.

—OPENING SENTENCES OF "NEW DIMENSIONS," A RADIO PROGRAM

HOSTED BY MICHAEL TOMS

THE SIX MOVEMENTS OF THE SPINE

Body Benefits:

➤ Rotates, flexes, extends, and aligns spine

➤ Stimulates spinal nerves

➤ Tones abdominals and back muscles

➤ Improves breathing

➤ Helps prevent incontinence

➤ Stimulates kidney function

➤ Activates peristalsis (digestion) and relieves constipation

➤ Increases circulation

➤ Brings fresh oxygen to musculoskeletal system

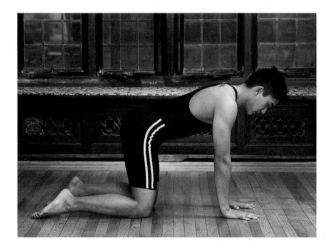

Zen is simply a voice crying, 'Wake up! Wake up!'

—MAHA

STHAVIRA

SANGHARAKSHITA

Let's begin:

MOVEMENTS 1 AND 2: THE CAT AND THE DOG

1. Begin down on your hands and knees in the Table position: your hands are directly underneath your shoulders, and your knees are directly underneath your hips. Keep your back flat, and your head in line with the rest of your spine. Imagine your back as a table on which you could balance tea cups.

2. Tuck your tailbone under and gently tilt your chin into your chest while you lift the middle and upper parts of the back toward the ceiling. Press the hips slightly forward. The spine is now rounded like a rainbow or a Halloween cat. This is called the Cat.

3. Tip the tailbone up, drop the belly toward the floor, and lift head and chin up toward the ceiling. You are not compressing the lower back; rather you are lengthening it. This position is the Dog.

4. Practice undulating the spine between the Cat and the Dog several times to loosen and warm the spinal column. As you begin to awaken the spine, allow the movements to be slow and mindful. There is no need to rush; allow yourself to luxuriate in the movements.

5. Establish a breathing rhythm. Inhale completely in one position, and exhale completely in the other. It doesn't matter which, as long as you are consistent.

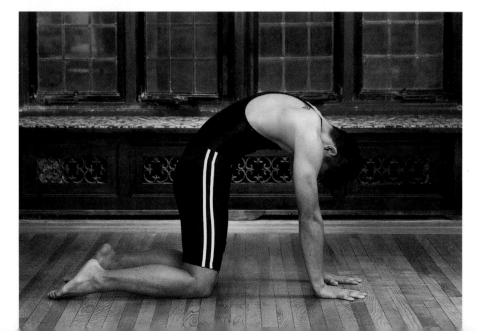

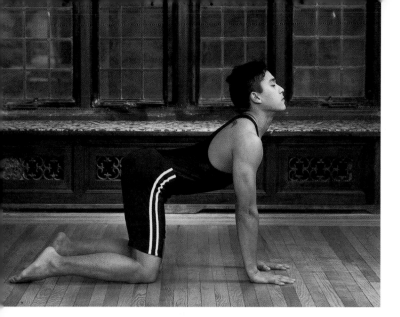

MOVEMENTS 3 AND 4: THE PUPPY DOG

1. In the Cat and Dog you flexed your spine up and down. In the next movements, you will move the spine from side to side.

2. Return to the Table position.

3. As you exhale, draw your right ear toward your right shoulder and bring your right shoulder toward your right hip. From an aerial view, your body will resemble a *C,* or a comma.

4. As you inhale, slowly come out of the comma position and return to the Table position.

5. As you exhale, bring your left ear toward your left shoulder and bring your left shoulder toward your left hip, once again forming a comma.

When to avoid this posture If you have had an abdominal hernia do not practice the Six Movements of the Spine. Avoid putting your head below your heart if you have glaucoma, detached retina, or uncontrolled high blood pressure. If you are beyond the third month of pregnancy, avoid the dog stretch, which hyper-extends the lower back.

Yoga Tip Your spine is an amazing creature! It can move in so many different directions. It can bend forward and backward, side to side, and it can twist, like wringing water out of a towel. Pay attention to your spine and treat it to this delightful series of movements—it will respond immediately! Close your eyes so you can develop an Awareness of the micro-movements. Begin to notice subtle details. Where does each movement initiate from? Watch how the rest of the spine follows the wave of this initial movement.

6. The movement between these two positions is smooth and continuous. Move with your breath in a slow, meditative way. The Puppy Dog is very subtle. If you sped up the movements, you would look like a dog wagging her tail.

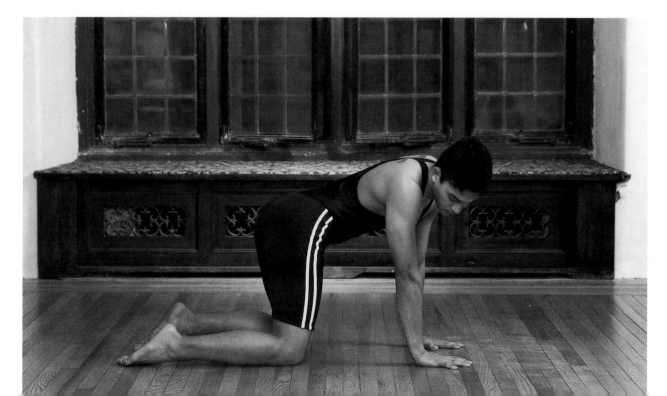

MOVEMENTS 5 AND 6: THREADING THE NEEDLE

1. Return to the Table position.

2. Lift the right hand and turn it over so that the palm is facing up with the fingertips pointing to the left. Imagine that the right arm is a needle.

3. "Thread" the right hand along the ground through the space between your left hand and the left knee. Slide the right arm as far as it can go, lowering your right ear and shoulder to the ground. Many beginners cannot rest their ears on the ground but instead lean on the forearm. The buttocks are now higher than the head.

4. Be careful not to strain your neck. Go only as far as is comfortable and allow yourself to relax completely in this position. Breathe!

5. For an additional stretch, lift your left arm overhead. Circle the left arm, rotating from the shoulder area. Spread the fingertips and explore the air around you, as if for the first time.

6. Bring the left arm down slowly and return the left hand to the floor. Press down into the left hand and lift the head and shoulders back up into the Table position.

7. Repeat Threading the Needle on the opposite side using the left arm as the needle.

8. Once you have completed the Six Movements of the Spine, sit quietly and notice the effects.

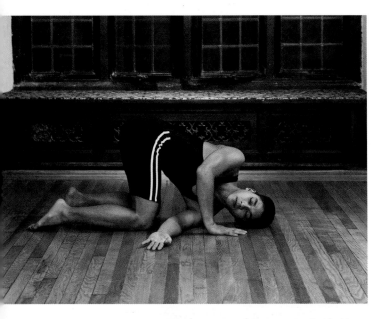

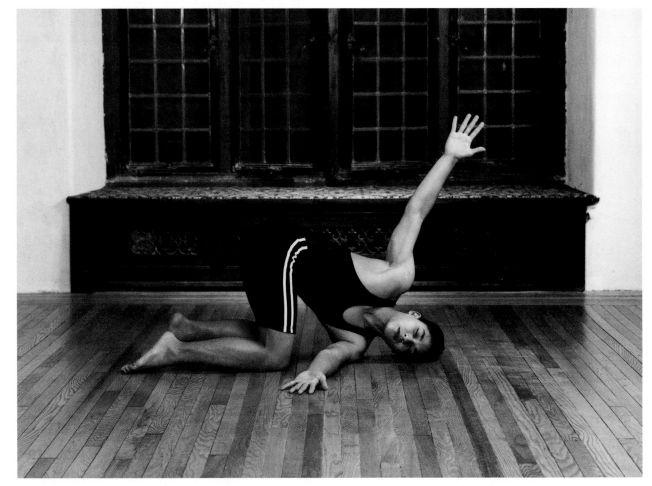

RUNNER'S STRETCH

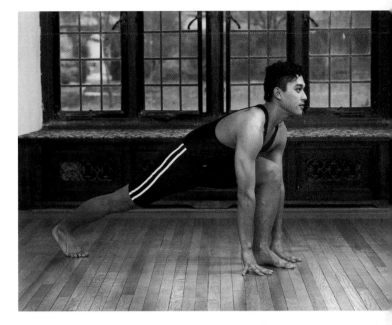

Body Benefits:

➤ Strengthens feet, ankles, knees, thighs, and hips

➤ Tones inner thigh muscles, buttocks, and hips

➤ Brings heat and energy into the body

➤ Stimulates digestion

➤ Stimulates circulation and respiration

Let's begin:

1. Come into the Table position. Your eyes can be either open or closed.

2. Lift the hips as you bring your right foot in between the two hands. Be sure that the knee is directly over the ankle and not hyperextended.

3. Press up onto the left toes and slide the left leg back until it is extended as straight as possible.

4. You may find that in order to hold this position you have lifted up onto your fingertips.

5. Press the left heel back toward the wall behind you and bring your attention into the sensations in the hips and legs.

6. Be sure not to collapse over the bent knee. Instead, maintain an Awareness of a lengthened spine with your head as a natural extension.

7. Hold for several breaths to your toleration level.

8. To release, lower the left knee to the ground and slide the right knee back to its original Table position.

9. Repeat steps 2–8 on the opposite side.

10. Once you have completed both sides, remain in the Table position or a comfortable seated position. Notice the sensations with complete Awareness of body and mind.

Yoga Tip Sometimes when we become aware, we don't like the visceral experience of fatigue, tightness, stiffness, discomfort, tension. Openness, vitality, looseness, and ease are more pleasurable to us. All of these feelings fall in the category of sensations. Remember: sensations are sensational—they simply mean that you are alive.

Runner's Stretch may seem simple, but use micromovements to find the sensations. As you press the heel toward the wall behind you, that whole leg will provide an arena for sensation exploration. The sensations may feel tingly, hot, or cold. Notice if they are tight or expansive, light or heavy. If the sensations had a color, what would it be? Become interested—you may notice that they move or change shape. Remember: within the *extra*ordinary is the ordinary!

I imagine how a chemist would write the equation for mindfulness: concentration + calm + equanimity + rapture + energy + investigation = mindfulness.

—SYLVIA BOORSTEIN, *DON'T JUST DO SOMETHING, SIT THERE*

FIVE-POINTED STAR

Body Benefits:

➤ Strengthens ankles, knees, hips, arms, back, shoulders, and neck

➤ Stimulates circulation and respiration

➤ Heats and energizes entire body

➤ Builds stability and endurance

➤ Activates digestion

Let's begin:

1. Begin in Proper Standing Alignment.

2. With conscious control, lift your arms out to the sides and up overhead. (See the Mountain Pose in the Confidence chapter.)

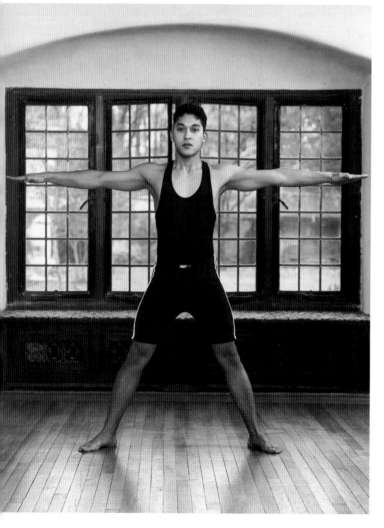

Yoga Tip Certainly to be aware of the infinite number of things present in our world would be exhausting and completely overwhelming. Yet there is so much happening in and around us of which we are often unaware. For example, we don't have to think about the heart for it to beat. Certain animals, such as bees, can perceive x-rays, ultraviolet light, and polarized light. Though invisible to us humans, we know they exist. Eskimos have attuned to the shades of difference in snow, and they have dozens of names for the delicate variations. When we expand our Awareness, a vast spectrum of knowing becomes available. With the door to the mind open and empty, we can be filled with grace.

3. Inhale. As you exhale, simultaneously separate your right foot from the left about a leg's length (or three feet) apart while lowering your arms out to your sides at shoulder height.

4. Point the toes in opposite directions and turn the palms down.

5. Engage all of yourself in this posture: extend your fingertips on each hand away from the center of your body, lift the thigh muscles up away from the knees, and relax the shoulders.

6. Hold to your toleration point, actively breathing into every cell in your body.

7. Bring your Awareness to all of the sensations. Feel yourself as a living miracle.

8. To come out of the posture, bring your right foot back to its original position while simultaneously drawing the arms back up overhead in the Mountain.

9. Exhale as you slowly extend and lower your arms back to their original position.

10. Take a moment to close your eyes and attune to your internal experience.

God lives in the details.

—SUFI EXPRESSION

HALF-MOON

Body Benefits:

➤ Rejuvenates adrenals

➤ Improves circulation

➤ Increases spinal flexibility

➤ Tones every centrally located muscle, including abdomen

➤ Firms waistline, hips, and buttocks

➤ Detoxifies kidneys, liver, and spleen

➤ Expands lung capacity

Yoga Tip Our sixth sense, or intuition, is another form of Awareness that can be strengthened. Men and particularly women are attracted to the power of the moon through all of her cycles. In the Half-Moon, imagine that you are moon bathing under a brightly lit starry sky. Use this deep symbol of the moon shining down on you to connect to the knowledge that has been available to people of all ages and cultures. In Shakti Gawain's *Living in the Light*, she says, "The intuitive mind . . . seems to have access to an infinite supply of information. It appears to be able to tap into a deep storehouse of knowledge and wisdom, the universal mind." Trust your hunches and your gut feelings. Call upon this rich inner guide as a way to access both practical resources as well as spiritual illumination.

Let's begin:

1. Start in Proper Standing Alignment. A variation for greater challenge: keep your feet together instead of directly under your hips.

2. Draw your arms out to the sides and overhead until the palms touch. Interlace your fingers, leaving the pointer fingers straight up, pressing against each other. This is known as steeple position. Keep your elbows straight and your arms beside your ears.

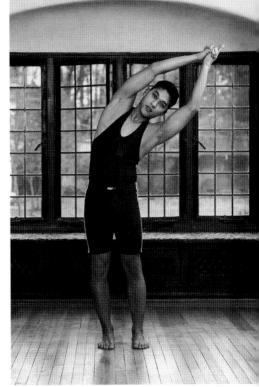

3. Relax the shoulders down even though the arms are overhead.

4. Inhale, and as you exhale, lift the torso up out of the waist. Press your right hip toward the right wall as you arch the upper body over to the left.

5. Your goal is not so much to arch the torso as far to the left as possible, but rather to keep your body aligned. Imagine that your body is between two panes of glass so that it remains in one plane. Keep your head between the arms and let your head follow the line of the spine in a natural extension.

6. Use your left hand to extend and lengthen the right arm.

7. As you hold for several breaths, breathe into the opening created on the right side of the body. Breathe into the spaces between the ribs to encourage expansion of lung capacity.

8. Inhale as you return to center. Remain with your fingers in steeple position and realign yourself.

9. Repeat steps 4–8 on the opposite side.

10. Once you have completed both sides, gently come out of the posture. If you feel steady, close your eyes as you release. Slowly separate the hands, first into the Mountain (Confidence chapter), and then gently lower the arms, extending them out to the sides. At shoulder height, turn your palms down, and continue the descent of your arms.

11. Take several deep breaths before moving on. Stand in Proper Standing Alignment and notice your experience at this moment.

FACE MASSAGE

Body Benefits:

➤ Increases circulation to face and scalp

➤ Relieves tension and stiffness in face

➤ Stimulates immune system

➤ Reduces stress and anxiety

➤ Creates sense of heightened well being

When to avoid this technique Check with your health care provider before massaging your face if you have a skin disorder.

Yoga Tip Your skin is the largest organ of your body. It weighs about six pounds and is around eighteen square feet in area! Yet, how often do you lovingly touch your body? Most of us take quick showers, not even giving thought to this miracle of skin that contains your essential being. We brush our teeth, slap on antiperspirant, and dress quickly. That's the extent of contact some of us have with the physical body. How sad!

Take two minutes to massage your face when you need a break at work or your eyes get tired. Massage your face as you would a loved one. Those few minutes can make a difference. With Face Massage, you both give and receive. Touch is healing.

Let's begin:

1. Be sure your hands are clean. Come into Proper Sitting Alignment with your eyes closed.

2. Rub your hands together vigorously to generate heat and energy in the palms and fingertips.

3. Using the soft part of the fingertips, place your three middle fingers at the meeting place of the eyebrows. Follow the line of the eyebrows with gentle but firm pressure until you reach the outer edges. Repeat this several times.

4. Moving up about a quarter of an inch at a time, continue this same motion from inside to outside until you reach your hairline. Imagine you are smoothing out any tension or worry lines.

5. Bring your fingertips to the bridge of your nose and press downward along your cheekbones as if you were wiping away tears. Repeat several times.

6. Draw your fingertips in front of your ears to your temples. Make small, steady circles.

7. Separate the lower jaw from the upper jaw slightly and practice this same circular massage technique between the two jaw bones. Try using the heels of your hands as you stimulate the soft spot between the two bones.

8. Press your fingertips into the center of the chin as if you were trying to create little dimples. With steady pressure, draw the fingertips up both sides of the cheeks, forming a giant smile.

9. Now grab the earlobes and pull them down. Travel up and around the edge of the ear, pulling it gently away from the head.

10. Slide your pointer fingertips behind each ear and rub the area where the ear meets the head.

11. Now give yourself a dry shampoo. Use all ten fingers to massage the scalp vigorously.

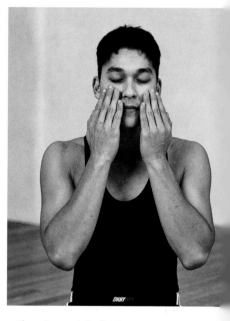

12. Let your fingers find any other areas around the face, neck or shoulders that require attention. Rub, knead, tap, or stroke them.

13. With curled fingers, tap gently on your chest below the collar bone (like Tarzan). Go ahead and say something when you are doing this to hear the vibration—it's fun!

14. When you feel complete, shake the hands out to release any tension that may have accrued. Notice the shifts that have occurred.

NATURAL BREATH

Body Benefits:

➤ Steadies emotions

➤ Revitalizes the body

➤ Creates clarity of mind

➤ Strengthens nervous system

➤ Purifies sinus and nasal passages

➤ Promotes sound sleep

Breathing Tip Practice the Natural Breath at times when you are relaxed. After you feel comfortable with it, use it before, during, or after periods of stress. As you develop your Awareness of the quality and rich texture of your breath, you gain access to the inner environment. A certain percentage of beginners will breathe backwards; that is, the belly contracts on the inhalation rather than expands. Our often stress-filled lives play a colossal role in changing our breathing patterns. Be patient yet persistent. This technique takes practice, but remember, it's called the Natural Breath and it is how we were born breathing. Recognizing the importance of increasing fresh oxygen in our system brings us halfway there. Oxygen is the most common element on the earth's crust, so enjoy its abundance in your life.

Let's begin:

1. Come into the Corpse Pose. If you have any lower-back discomfort or difficulty feeling the movement of your breath, bend your knees. Separate the feet wider apart than your hips and let the knees rest against each other.

2. Focus your attention on your abdomen and the area around your belly button. Place your hands there.

3. Inhale slowly and deeply through your nose with the mouth closed. Feel and imagine your belly expanding up toward the ceiling like an inflating balloon.

4. Exhale slowly and fully. Imagine the balloon deflating. Feel your belly sinking back toward your spine.

5. Repeat steps 3 and 4 for several minutes as you become aware of the breath moving in and out of your body.

6. Notice the peaceful effect of this exercise on your body and mind.

Breathe consciously . . . because that is life—not whether you drive a BMW or pay the rent on time. Life is the state of being, not doing. That state of being is enhanced and intensified through breath.

—IYANLA VANZANT, AUTHOR OF *VALUE IN THE VALLEY: A BLACK WOMAN'S GUIDE THROUGH LIFE'S DILEMMA,* FROM "NEW DIMENSIONS" PUBLIC RADIO INTERVIEW

P R I V A T E   " I "   I N V E S T I G A T I O N

Yoga Tip This relaxation technique invites you to attend the celebration of your life. You can practice it time and time again to return to a mindful appreciation of your unique being.

There are two parts to this exercise. You can do them separately or together. As a variation to Part II, work with a partner and outline each others' bodies on a giant piece of paper as you rest in the Corpse Pose. Then, using crayons or magic markers, color in the places that feel tight, tense, loose, and so on. If your stomach feels balled up in knots, draw knots in that area. Choose colors that represent the feelings present in your body. You might choose green to show an area in which Awareness is growing. Black might be just right for places from which you feel disconnected.

Let's begin:

Part I

1. Begin standing as you normally do without trying to do it right. Allow your eyes to close.

2. Take several breaths, inhaling through the nose and exhaling with a sigh through an open mouth. Imagine that you are a private detective looking for clues. The being that you are investigating is yourself. Without judgment, begin to explore.

3. Begin at your feet. Feel both feet on the ground. Without looking, feel the direction that your toes point: out to the sides, slightly inward, or straight out in front of you?

4. Notice if you have a tendency to lean more on one foot than the other or if you are balanced. If you do lean, which foot carries more weight? Do not shift around. Simply notice.

5. Become aware of where you place the weight on your feet. Do you lean more on your toes or on the balls of your feet? Do you lean more toward the inside or outside edges of the feet? Perhaps you feel that you are equally centered.

6. Bring your attention up to your pelvis. Imagine that it is a large bowl. The bottom of the bowl rests at your groin and the top opens at your hip bones. Imagine that this bowl is filled with water. Does the water stay in the bowl or spill out in front, behind, to the right or left? Notice your torso as you breathe into it. Does the torso grow straight up from the basket of your pelvic bowl? Does it lean in front of the bowl? Behind?

7. Become conscious of where your arms rest. Are they touching any other part of your body? What about your hands and fingers? Do you clutch them or are they loose?

8. Shift your attention up to your shoulders. Are the shoulders even or is one higher than the other? If so, which one? Is this the shoulder that you carry bags or purses on? Is this the shoulder of your dominant hand?

9. Move your Awareness up to your head. Does the head sit directly atop your shoulders? Does it jut out in front of the shoulders or extend behind them? Does the chin lift up toward the ceiling? Is it tucked in toward the chest?

10. Having gathered all of this information, open your eyes for a moment and shake the body around. Now, bring yourself into Proper Standing Alignment. Go back and review the questions in steps 2–11. Has anything changed? What are the differences and similarities?

Part II

1. In slow motion, bring your body down onto the floor in the Corpse Pose with the eyes closed. Bend the knees with your feet flat on the ground and place your hands on your belly.

2. Feel the detail of your breath. Notice how the hands rise with the inhalation and fall with the exhalation. Remain focused on this simple movement for a few moments.

3. Notice the weight of your hands on your belly. Notice the weight of your clothes on your skin.

4. Bring your attention to your face. Is your forehead wrinkled? Relax it. Let the eyelids form a protective layer over your eyes without squinting. Let go of any tension in the cheeks. Slightly separate the upper jaw from the lower jaw.

5. Straighten the legs so that the whole backside of your body rests on the ground.

6. Now mentally divide your body in half, from the top of the head through the middle of the forehead, nose, mouth, right through the torso and to the groin. Imagine that you could exist only in the right half of your body. What does it feel like? Is it tight or open? Does it have a texture? A color?

7. Now shift over into the left half. What does it feel like? Is it tight or open? Does it have a texture? A color? Now, put the two halves back together again. Is one side heavier? Lighter?

8. In your imagination, divide the body with an imaginary line down through the ear, the shoulder, the hip, and the side of the leg to the ankle.

9. For a moment, live only in the front half of your body. What does it feel like? Is it tight or open? Does it have a texture? A color? Now shift to the back side and notice how it feels. Is it tight or open? Does it have a texture? A color? Mentally bring the front and back together again.

10. Do an internal scan of your body to locate places that are still holding on, tense, or tight. If you find any, breathe into them as if your breath could visit these places and soothe them.

11. Now as you scan the body, find places that feel safe, open, comfortable, and relaxed. Spend some time there exploring them.

12. Deepen your breath now, feeling the body in contact with the floor. Notice which parts of the back side of the body are actually touching the floor: the heels, the backs of the legs, the back, the buttocks. Notice how the back of the neck and head are resting on the floor.

13. Gently roll over onto one side, hugging the knees up toward your chest. How do you feel at this moment? Draw your body back up into a comfortable seated position. Send a message of reverence to your body for all the ways that it has served you.

CREATE YOUR OWN POSTURE FOR AWARENESS

Let's begin:

1. Come into Proper Standing Alignment with your eyes closed. Take several long and deep breaths.

2. Become aware of your hands: each finger, your palms, the knuckles.

3. Begin to play with the endless variety of shapes you can make with your hands and fingers. Slowly stretch the palms, contract into fists, make claws with some fingers but not others.

4. As you grow more and more absorbed in the miracle of your hands, expand the slow motion movement to involve your arms, shoulders, and upper torso.

5. Let the stretches naturally move into the pelvis, legs, and feet.

6. When you find a position that captures your attention, stop and hold it, breathing fully.

7. What does this posture feel like? What is happening in your mind?

8. You may wish to draw or write about this posture. Create an affirmative statement of your commitment to being present. Confirm your belief by repeating it aloud or silently when you engage this posture. Name your posture and add it to your series on Awareness.

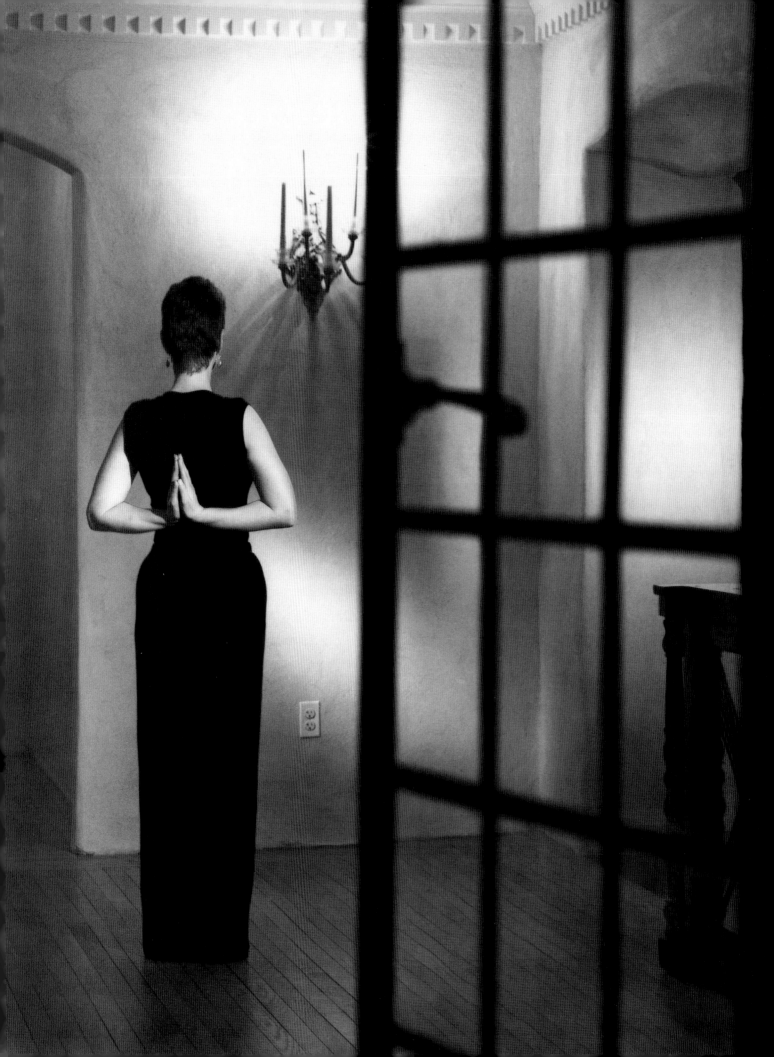

ACCEPTANCE

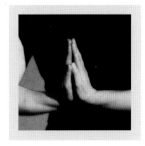

If you want to go to California but you're stuck in New Jersey, wishing otherwise won't bring you any closer to the West Coast. By wanting a situation to be other than it is, we drain our vital energy, tying it up with a knot of resistance.

Every day we get messages from the media that we are lacking. No matter what we've got or who we are, it's never good enough. When we constantly desire things that we don't have, we feel deficient, anxious, and jealous. The fact that we don't own a brand new car every year is not the cause of our discontent. *Believing* that we are deficient is the problem.

It's easy to accept circumstances when things are going our way. But many of us are perfectionists, and everything we do must be of the finest quality or we won't do it at all. We need to begin practicing the art of *self*-Acceptance. Try a new sport, game, or recipe. Adopt a noncompetitive attitude and let yourself be a beginner. See how many mistakes you can make! If you miss the ball or create an inedible meal, let it be okay. The world will not end if your team loses or your cornbread has the consistency of a brick. Being partial only to *familiar* paths in life leads us down the road to prejudice. Bias, on a large or small scale, causes injury to both parties.

Once we accept the diversity within ourselves, including our strengths and weaknesses, we can begin to accept the multidimensional world. We don't have to like everyone, but learning tolerance

is crucial to maintaining a peaceful world. Ageism, sexism, homophobia, and racism are as prevalent as the common cold, but far more fatal. The paradoxical attitude "I am better than you," or its flip side "You are superior to me," puts bars around our humanity. By not accepting or denying the things we dislike in ourselves, we create disease and segregation from our inner being.

In order to achieve a sense of wholeness, we must embrace not only our light, but also our darkness. How often have the so-called negative incidents in our lives brought us our greatest lessons? Seen as gifts, all of our experiences hold within them valuable lessons. Both contemporary psychology as well as traditional religious stories speak of the healing made possible by embracing the shadow.

Christianity helps its believers bear their own crosses. Saint Francis of Assisi's most popular prayer starts with a surrender to God, "Lord, make me an instrument of your peace." The ultimate role model, Jesus, proclaimed, "Thy will be done." As we come to accept that which we cannot change, we understand the power of surrender. Another version of this surrender to a higher power is found in the twelve-step recovery programs. Step two reads "Come to believe that a Power greater than ourselves could restore us to sanity." Denial is part of the insanity of addiction. We all have our own denial disease, which is the antithesis of Acceptance. The "Power" could be anything you want. It might be your own god, nature, or the higher self within you.

The world is not made up of fairy-tale figures. No one is entirely good witch or bad witch. Expecting ourselves to fit only one mold is harmful. Yoga, meaning union, helps to heal the splits and divisions that we create within ourselves.

Life *isn't* fair. We are all wounded in some way—whether it be relationships, health, money, or another issue. We must not use our own feelings of fear, lack, or disappointment to create an environment of hostility and unwelcome for ourselves or others.

Practicing yoga will bring you face to face with Acceptance. There will be times when your body will not be able to hold a posture or when your uncooperative hamstrings won't stretch. Some days you'll set aside time for yoga to help you reduce stress, and it will bring you more in touch with your anger and resentment. Your breath can help you embrace and integrate these missing pieces so that you will experience a deeper sense of wholeness.

Trust that by putting your body into different positions you explore the many levels of being that a human can be confronted with. In doing so, you validate and affirm the very nature of existence. Acceptance is not passivity or giving up. Rather, it is an active willingness to face all aspects of our humanness. Acceptance is an acknowledgment of what is and an opportunity to find meaning in it.

Postures for Acceptance Explore the Seated Angle, the Sphinx, the Bridge, and the Straight-Legged Runner's Stretch as a prayer for self-Acceptance. Standing Yoga Mudra is the ultimate symbol of surrender to the highest in yourself and others.

Breathing Lesson for Acceptance Your belief in yourself will grow strong with the I AM breath. You confirm your existence as a rightful being in this world.

Meditation for Acceptance Childspirit Meditation reminds you to accept the vulnerable little person inside of yourself.

SEATED ANGLE

Body Benefits:

➤ Tones, stretches, and lengthens spine and back of legs

➤ Improves digestion and relieves constipation

➤ Stimulates pancreas, liver, gall-bladder, spleen, bladder, gonads

➤ Increases circulation, especially in pelvic region

➤ Helps regulate menstrual irregularities

➤ Helps irrigate kidneys

When to avoid this posture Practice with caution if you suffer from sciatica or have stiff, weak back muscles. Do not put pressure on the belly if you are pregnant.

Yoga Tip In this posture, most of us can easily find our edge. It's the place where the inner thighs scream "Wow!"; the lower back shrieks "Hey!"; and the mind yelps "Help!" This edge (before you get to pain, but still challenging) is where we learn about ourselves; it is a powerful teacher. Be with yourself in a loving way even when discomfort arises. Not putting any effort into the pose at all is like ignoring a child crying for help. Forcing the stretch is like pushing away a hurt child. Exploring the edge is loving the child.

Let's begin:

1. Come into Proper Sitting Alignment with your legs straddled out as far as is comfortable. Flex your toes back toward your face.

2. Place your hands in front of your body and, with a flat back, begin to lean the torso forward slowly. You can either leave your arms out-stretched in front of you (for more support), or

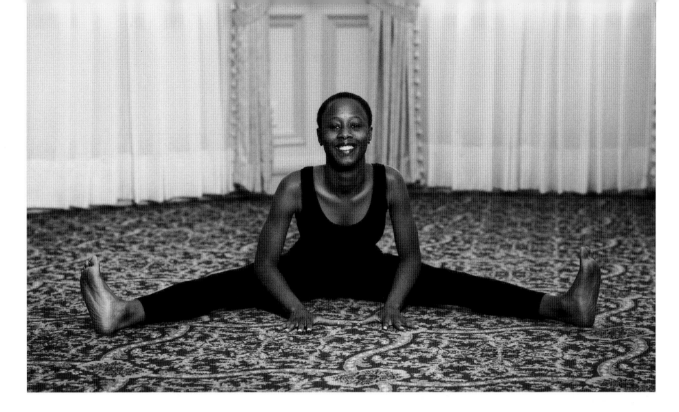

place your hands on either leg and let them slide down the legs as you come forward. Pause, hold, and breathe deeply every inch or so.

3. Don't let your feet and legs roll inward. Be sure to keep your knees pointing up toward the ceiling. When you come down to the place where you feel a definite stretch (but not strain), lower your chin to your chest and round the spine.

4. If you are pushing yourself beyond your limits, back off the stretch somewhat and hold here. Accepting your limits will make the experience more fulfilling.

5. Hold for five to ten breaths, maintaining an inward focus.

6. To release, bring your hands back in front of you for support and feel the sitting bones pressing into the floor. Roll up the spine, stacking the vertebrae one on top of the other.

7. Slowly draw your legs together in front of you and bounce them slightly to relieve any residual tension that may be present.

8. Sit with the eyes closed as you integrate the Seated Angle.

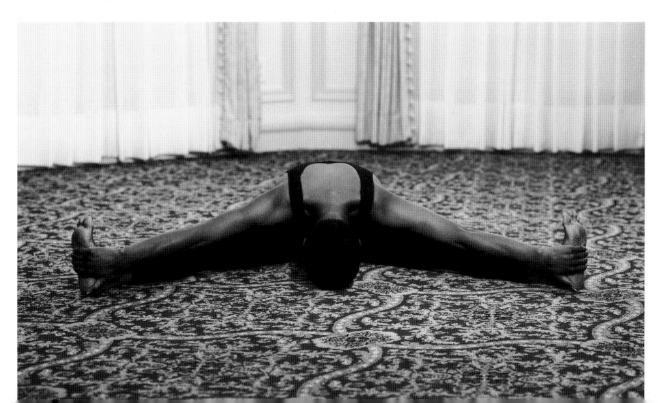

SPHINX

Body Benefits:

➤ Heats and invigorates body

➤ Opens lungs and expands rib cage and chest

➤ Delivers fresh blood and oxygen to pelvis and reproductive organs

➤ Rejuvenates kidneys

➤ Improves digestive functioning and relieves constipation

➤ Relieves menstrual and menopausal discomfort

➤ Strengthens back muscles

➤ Tones, aligns, strengthens, and flexes spine

➤ Relaxes nervous system

When to avoid this posture Do not practice the Sphinx after the third month of pregnancy. If you have suffered recent abdominal surgery or abdominal inflammation, avoid the Sphinx.

Yoga Tip Enjoy this milder version of the Cobra. To gain the same benefits, you don't always have to bring each posture to its fullest expression. This concept is often an epiphany to many of us. Sometimes you will need to accept the limitations of your current situation. Respect the diversity of your physical experience from day to day. Cultivate a sense of gratitude for the capabilities that you *do* have.

Let's begin:

1. Begin on the floor on your belly. Rest your forehead on the ground. Spread your fingers apart and place your hands underneath your shoulders with your elbows as close to the body as possible.

2. Draw the legs together if you are able. Imagine that you can zip them up from the toes to the buttocks. Keep the buttocks squeezed and press the pelvic triangle (the two hip bones and the pubic bone) down into the floor.

3. Wiggle your torso out of the waist. Keep the shoulders relaxed and press the crown of the head away from the feet.

4. Lift the torso beginning with the forehead, nose, chin, and finally the neck, shoulders, and upper chest.

5. Slide your palms forward until your elbows are directly underneath your shoulders and you are balanced on the forearms. Be aware of your shoulders taking a ride up toward the ears. If you notice this, press them down through the back.

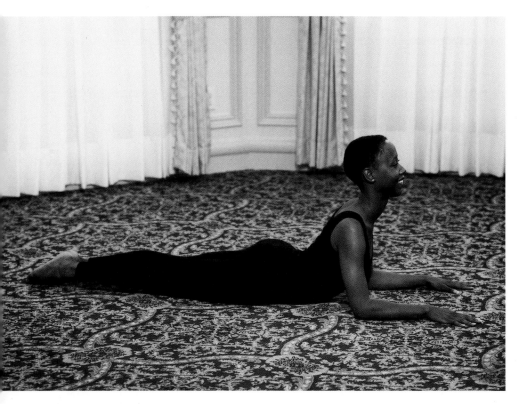

YOGA STORY FOR ACCEPTANCE: LYNNE DAVIES

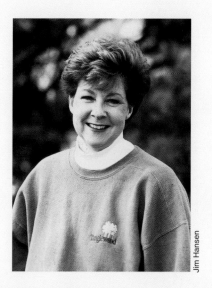

Jim Hansen

When Lynne Davies found out that she had inherited adult-onset diabetes and needed to take insulin, she knew she had to do something to help herself deal with it.

I was a wreck. My whole endocrine system was off. My blood pressure was really high and I was extremely vulnerable. I had a little bit of the "why me" syndrome, but mostly I was very resistant and scared to death of the idea of giving myself insulin shots. I hate needles!

I knew I needed to do something to get through this very frightening time. I brainstormed my choices. I could have gone to a therapist, the gym, or for regular massage. I chose yoga because when I had taken a class several years earlier, it brought me deeply in touch with myself. But this time yoga was more than just beneficial—it was life changing.

I needed an anchor and yoga stabilized me at this crucial time. Connecting with my breath gave my mind a chance to stop running. It helped to calm and center me. Although it was a very difficult time in my life, yoga gently brought me in touch with the truth of my reality. Yoga teaches you that how you breathe is directly related to how you feel. As I consistently focused on deep, slow breathing, I could handle my emotions better. Instead of trying to change my situation, I breathed into the myriad of unsettling feelings I was having—and they became less overwhelming. Yoga also helped reassure me of the decisions I was making. It brought me to a clearer and higher level of Acceptance of a disease that I will live with for the rest of my life.

Now I give myself insulin shots every day. I'm at the point where I'm even *grateful* for the glucometer—a little machine that measures the level of glucose in the blood. Unlike a urine sample, which is old information, this is a sophisticated piece of equipment that gives me a reading in forty-five seconds with just a prick of the finger. This is the kind of advance that my father (who also had diabetes) didn't get to use. I have the luxury of using it between four and eight times a day.

Like yoga, the glucometer is now part of my daily ritual—and an integral part of my life.

6. Keep your gaze fixed on a point on the wall at eye level. Maintain open and deep breathing. Remain in the Sphinx for as long as you comfortably can.

7. When you are ready to release, keep the buttocks squeezed and begin to roll back down from the middle belly all the way down to the forehead. Slide your palms back toward your hips and rest them on the ground.

8. Once you have returned to the original position, turn your head to one side, close your eyes, release the squeeze in the buttocks, and rest. You may want to windshield-wipe the lower legs from side to side, or in and out (in either the American or the European version).

9. To counterbalance the back bending, fold your hips back to your heels into the Child Pose.

10. Take several moments to integrate the benefits of the Sphinx into your being.

BRIDGE

Body Benefits:

- ➤ Stimulates functioning of thyroid gland and endocrine system
- ➤ Relieves fatigue
- ➤ Strengthens back and shoulder muscles
- ➤ Activates kidney functioning
- ➤ Strengthens and stretches abdominals
- ➤ Improves complexion
- ➤ Promotes greater spinal flexibility
- ➤ Helps relieve bed sores
- ➤ Tones legs and buttocks

Yoga Tip One of the most healing ways to cultivate Acceptance is through forgiveness. Consider the people (including yourself), circumstances, and events toward which you harbor resentment. Imagine that your body is a bridge leading you from struggle to forgiveness. Recall what you may be ready to let go of as you hold this posture. When you release the pose, let your body merge slowly into the "water" of the floor, the symbol of cleansing and purification. Allow the water to dissolve grudges, resistance, and stubbornness. Surrender into the accepting arms of water and feel your energy being replenished.

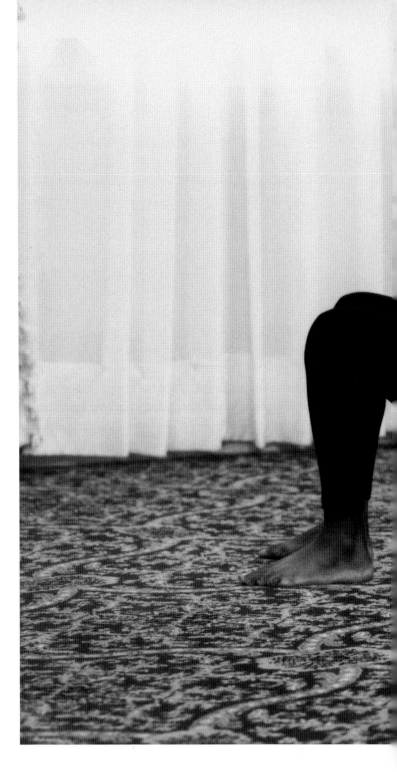

Let's begin:

1. Begin in a position lying on your back with your knees bent and feet flat on the floor. The feet are parallel and hip width apart, with the arms resting by your sides, palms down.

2. Squeeze the buttocks as you roll the lower, middle, and upper back off the floor, lifting the hips slowly in the air. Press your belly and the pelvic triangle up toward the ceiling.

3. Once your hips are as high as possible, walk your shoulders together to form padding.

4. If you can, clasp your hands underneath your back on the floor. Or, simply use the arms beneath you to support your weight.

5. As you hold the Bridge, breathe into the whole front side of the body, from the belly all the way to the upper chest. Keep your chin tucked in and heart open as you breathe into it.

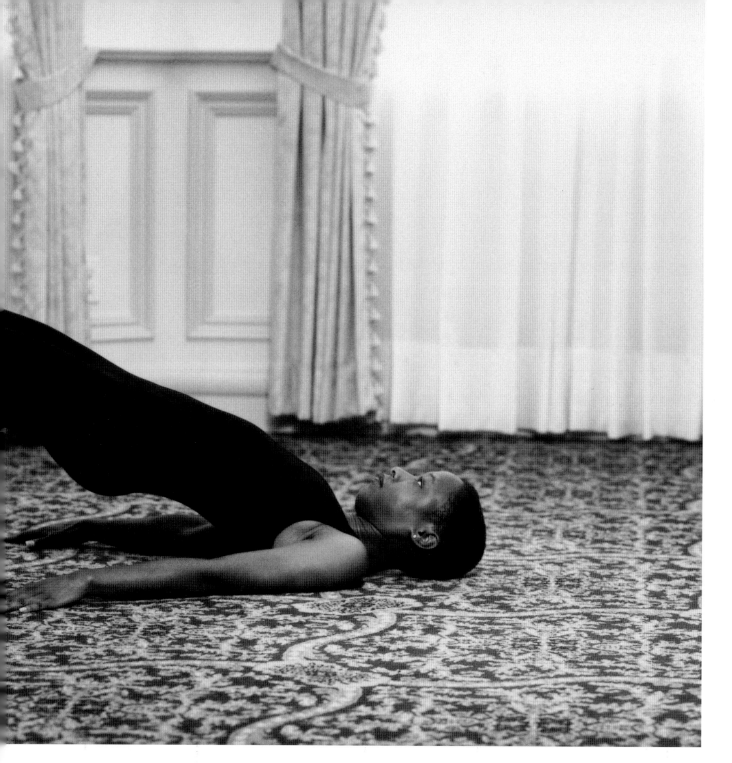

6. To release, walk the shoulders carefully back to their original position. Separate your hands and place them on the floor palms down on either side of the hips.

7. Roll down the spine from the upper to the middle to the lower back. Return the hips to the ground and exhale with a sigh, "Aaah. . . ." Notice the effects and benefits of the Bridge integrating into your physical and etheric body.

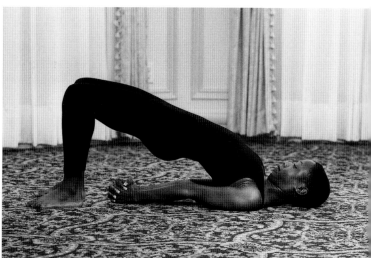

STRAIGHT-LEGGED RUNNER'S STRETCH

Body Benefits:

➤ Relieves stiffness in legs and hips

➤ Improves spinal flexibility

➤ Tones abdominal organs

➤ Opens chest and shoulders, facilitating breathing

➤ Oxygenates pancreas, gallbladder, kidneys, spleen, liver

➤ Brings nourishment to facial skin and scalp

➤ Improves memory, concentration, and relieves some headaches

When to avoid this posture Do not practice if you have eye or ear ailments such as weak eye capillaries, glaucoma, conjunctivitis, or any inflammation. Other contraindications include shoulder problems or uncontrolled high blood pressure. Proceed with caution if you are pregnant, have sciatica, or have weak or stiff back muscles. As a variation, stand facing a wall. Proceed until step 3; then, with a flat back (parallel to the floor), reach forward and press the palms against the wall.

Yoga Tip Before practicing this pose, take a moment to look at yourself in the mirror. Practice the art of self-Acceptance by seeing yourself exactly as you are. Imagine the eyes of Acceptance looking at you through your own eyes. Begin with your face and travel down to your feet as you find the parts that you like while accepting the others. Remember how lucky you are to have a functioning body. Now, come into this posture with reverence for yourself.

Yoga is about progress, not perfection.
—ALICIA SCOTT, YOGA STUDENT

Let's begin:

1. Begin in Proper Standing Alignment. Separate your feet a leg's length apart as you draw your arms up overhead. Bring the palms together, fingers pointing up and thumbs crossed.

2. Pivot your body ninety degrees to your left so that both feet are facing the same direction, left leg in front. Keep the shoulders relaxed by drawing them down into the back. Maintain your awareness of a lengthened spine.

3. Hinge at the hips with a flat back and extend the torso forward slowly. Come into a jackknife position with your torso parallel to the floor. The arms continue to frame the ears. If this is as far as you can go, lower your arms and let them rest on your front leg. Bend the front knee as much as you need to in order to bring your forehead to the knee.

4. If you are able to go further, continue to extend the arms forward and all the way to the ground, placing the hands on either side of your feet or holding the leg. Bring the chin to the chest and the forehead to the knee. Again, you may want to bend the front knee in order to do so.

5. Whether you are at step 3 or 4, keep the breath moving fluidly even as you feel your belly pressing against your thigh. Hold for up to ten breaths.

6. To release, extend your arms back out alongside your ears with palms together. Bend the forward knee. With a flat back, push off to an upright position with the palms overhead. It may be helpful to roll back up the spine, stacking the vertebrae one on top of the other.

7. Pivot back to face forward and repeat steps 1–6 on the opposite side.

8. Once you have completed both sides, place the feet together. Slowly lower the arms down to your sides.

9. If you are at all dizzy, leave your eyes open. Otherwise, close your eyes and take several deep breaths to integrate the effects of Straight-Legged Runner's Stretch.

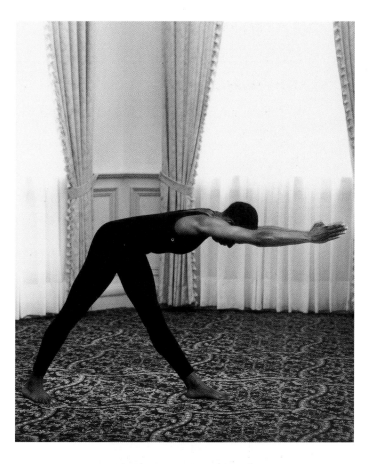

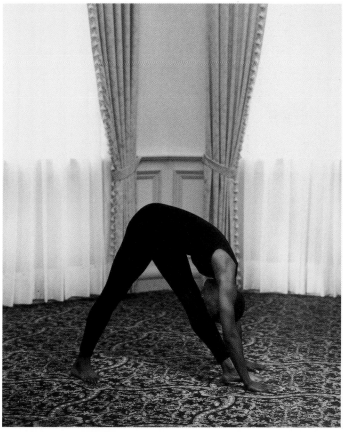

STANDING YOGA MUDRA

Body Benefits:

➤ Creates internal experience of self-love and humility

➤ Strengthens leg muscles

➤ Brings a fresh supply of blood to brain

➤ Nourishes facial skin, scalp, hair roots

➤ Opens and expands chest

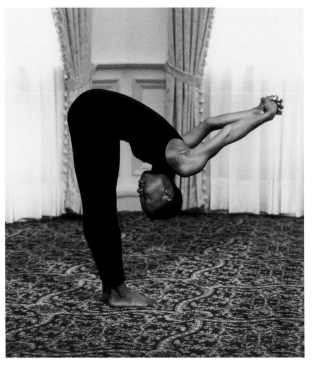

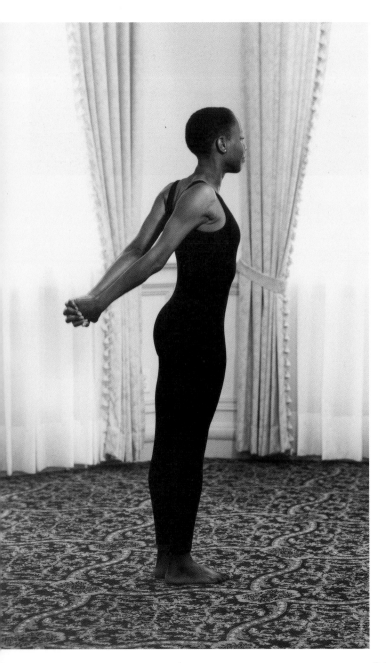

When to avoid this posture People with recent or chronic shoulder injury should avoid Standing Yoga Mudra, but as a variation can practice the Rag Doll.

If you have detached retina or any inflammation of the eyes or ears, uncontrolled high blood pressure, a history of heart disease or stroke, or are pregnant, keep your head above your heart. Do not allow your head to fall below your heart in Standing Yoga Mudra, but instead follow the variation described in step 4.

Yoga Tip Standing Yoga Mudra is the universal symbol of yoga. As you place your head below your heart, you symbolically bow to the spirit within yourself and others. Mudra means "a sealing posture." While in Standing Yoga Mudra, seal in your inner light, inner peace, and goodness.

This is a beautiful posture. My classes sometimes stand in a circle in Standing Yoga Mudra, simultaneously bowing to ourselves and each other. Students celebrating their birthdays are invited to stand in the middle of the circle as a powerful way to receive birthday blessings.

Let's begin:

1. Assume Proper Standing Alignment.

2. Lift your arms out in front of you, with your palms facing away from each other. Bring your hands behind you until they meet at the base of your spine.

3. Interlace your fingers. Squeeze the shoulder blades together, pressing the palms into each other. Feel your chest opening.

4. On an exhalation, with a flat back, bend the torso forward from the hips. Let your head hang down. Your fingers will stay interlaced, though the palms may have separated.

   Variation for those who must avoid this posture: Maintain a flat back parallel to the ground. Keep your head in line with your spine; do not drop your head below your heart. Do not follow step 5. Instead, remain in this position for a few deep breaths and skip to step 7.

5. Lift your hands overhead as far as they can go. Our model, Alicia, is extremely flexible. Your arms may stretch only slightly away from the body. Without locking the knees, keep the legs straight and release the head, so that the neck is relaxed.

6. Take several full, deep breaths in this posture.

7. To release, slowly bend the knees and tuck in the tailbone. Keep your palms clasped as you roll the body back up, stacking the vertebrae one on top of the other.

8. Once you are back in an upright position, if you are at all light-headed from the blood rushing to your head, keep your eyes open. If you're not dizzy, close your eyes. *Slowly* separate your hands, and allow them to float back around in front of you in slow motion.

9. Stand in stillness for a moment to receive and integrate the benefits of this posture.

There is so much relief when we learn to accept what is—all of what is—and get on with acting on it to make constructive changes.

—DAVID K. REYNOLDS, PH.D.

CREATE YOUR OWN POSTURE FOR ACCEPTANCE

Let's begin:

1. Practice the formal postures before you begin.

2. Come into any starting position that feels good to you. You can stand, sit, or lie down.

3. Close your eyes and deeply connect with your breath.

4. Feel, notice, and observe areas of the body that are open, loose, and relaxed. Now feel, notice, and observe any areas of tightness, tension, fatigue, or discomfort. Allow them to be without trying to resist them.

5. Imagine that each of these limitations is a precious child for whom you are caring. With respect for these sensations, begin to explore movements that are comfortable and gentle.

6. Work around these limits as if they were sacred jewels. Know that you are the caretaker of these treasures that bring you closer to your humanness.

7. In your exploration of ways to love these sensations, you may find positions that you wish to hold. When one feels particularly sacred to you, stay there and breathe deeply.

8. Become deeply attuned to the limitations of your body. Try having a chat with them. Ask them what they are doing there, how they serve you, and what they need. Ask them how you can transform them into possibilities for expanding your consciousness.

9. After you have finished dialoguing, form an affirmation that supports you as you nurture the development of Acceptance. Repeat this belief or prayer when you are in your posture.

10. You may wish to draw or write about this posture. Give it a name. Add it to your Acceptance sequence or find a new one each time to accommodate your current situation.

The spirit of yoga is the spirit of self-acceptance in the present moment. The idea is to explore your limits gently, lovingly, with respect for your body. It is not to try to break through your body's limits because you want to look better or fit into your bathing suit better next summer.

—JON KABAT-ZINN, PH.D.

I AM BREATH

Yoga Tip Both Eastern and Western traditions incorporate prayers that use the affirming and accepting phrase "I am," or a closely related expression. Within the great mystery of life, you can deeply affirm your essence with this ritual act of Acceptance. As you embrace the reality that *you are*, and *we all are*, you are better able to feel your communion with the sacred.

Let's begin:

1. Come into Proper Sitting Alignment with your eyes closed.

2. Take several long, deep, slow breaths.

3. Focus on the length of the inbreath as well as the quality of the outbreath.

4. In your head, hear the word *I* on the inhalation.

5. In your head, hear the word *am* on the exhalation.

6. When you exhale, let the word *am* be slightly longer than the inhalation. Let the *am* sound like a hum inside of your head.

7. Stay absorbed with these two words as they merge and meld with your breath. Use this breath to help you embrace and integrate any missing pieces of the whole you: anger, resentment, fear, sadness, and so on.

8. Continue with this same pattern for three to five minutes. You may wish to hum, speak, or sing these words aloud.

9. When you feel complete, allow the words to fall away. Return to simply watching the breath.

10. Sit in stillness and in silence for several minutes. Notice the deeply integrating feeling as you sense your whole self interconnected in divine union. Slowly allow your eyes to open.

I feel like I never had time to be a kid. I didn't have time for myself, time to relax. Through yoga, I realize how important it is to do both.

—HEATHER SOCCIO,
YOGA STUDENT

Yoga helped me realize that I was looking for the answers to my problems outside of myself. And that was my problem. I needed to look within.

—DARIN OLSEN,
YOGA STUDENT

CHILDSPIRIT MEDITATION

Yoga Tip Think of yourself as a Russian nesting doll. These dolls that fit snugly each inside another represent you at different ages. The littlest one symbolizes you as a baby or earlier. The next-larger one is you as a toddler. Several dolls bigger stands for the seven-year-old you, and so on. It's as if all of the people you have been still live inside you underneath the layers of who you are today. Nurturing a safe space for the younger yous creates an attitude of receptivity for the big one that you are today.

Let's begin:

1. Come into the Corpse Pose. You may wish to drape a blanket over yourself for warmth. Take several deep, relaxing breaths.

2. In your mind's eye, see yourself as a child. Choose an image that comes to mind readily, without judging or censoring it. You may recall a photograph or old family movie. It may be a joy-filled image of a birthday party, holiday celebration, or vacation.

3. Whether the image and age that you choose has happy or painful associations, stay present with it and with the emotions that arise.

4. Imagine that you are watching an old movie. Begin to explore the image further; let it come to life. As an observer, take note of what you look, act, and sound like. Who else is present? What are you doing in this setting? What is the emotional climate of this particular scene?

5. Now focus more deeply on the child that is you. Notice your nuances, distinct features, and body language. What do you, as a child, need?

6. See yourself now *at your current age* entering the scenario. Allow the child to see you. As the adult, what might you say to this little person? Knowing all that you know, approach the child gently and do or say whatever feels right. You might hug the child or offer words of encouragement, advice, or love.

7. Let the child know that you accept her in every way. Welcome her into your heart as you embrace the little one that you once were. Spend several moments together with your child self. Seek to remove any barriers that may thwart your connection.

8. Look deeply into the eyes of this child and recall that you are the same being. Offer your belief and Acceptance of her either through words, a loving look, or any other way that works for you.

9. Feel the spirit of your unified self. What does it feel like to host a warm and generous reception for this part of you in the spaciousness of your vast heart?

10. Say the final thing that you wish to say to your young child right now, knowing that you can connect with her whenever you want.

11. When you feel complete, say good-bye. Offer this child the gift of knowing that you are always available to her. Take her presence back with you. Know that she is the childlike spirit that resides within.

12. Deepen your breath, feeling yourself back in the room at the present moment. Inhale and draw in the validation for all that you have been and all that you are yet to become. As you exhale, let go into the present moment without judgment.

13. Know that in any circumstance in your life you can offer your adult self the same kind of Acceptance that you gave to this child.

14. Gently roll over on your side into the fetal position. You probably spent most of your time in this position when you were in your mother's womb. Savor the comfort of being curled up safe and sound.

15. With great care, as though you were an infant or child waking up from a soothing nap, roll up into a comfortable seated position. Become aware of your inner experience. Move gently into the rest of your day.

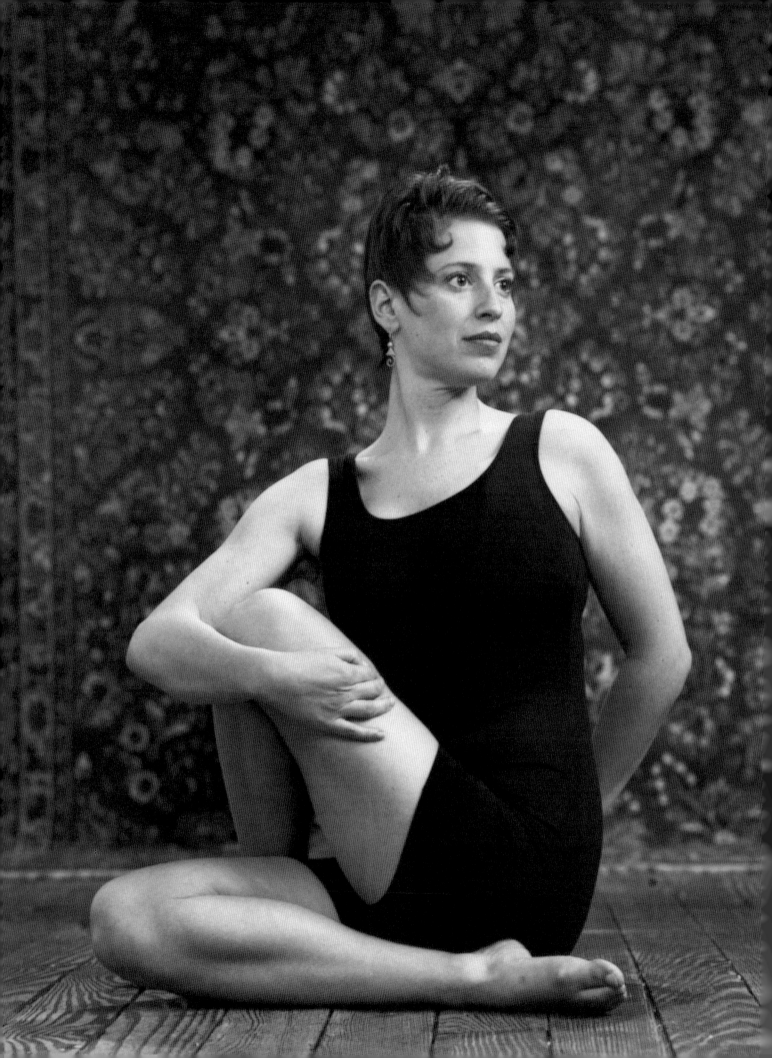

FOCUS

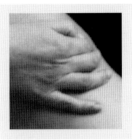

Imagine yourself in the audience of a live television show. As you look onto the stage, your attention is drawn to many aspects of the show: actors, scenery, costumes, and lighting. However, if the stage is completely dark except for a spotlight illuminating a single performer, your attention is focused. Yoga encourages you to do the spotlighting yourself.

Similarly, when your own television screen is out of Focus, you try to make it clearer. Fuzzy, blurry, vague pictures are distracting at best and disturbing at worst. You need not only clear, sharply defined, and distinct images, you also need to develop a deep commitment to their purpose in a busy internal and external world.

Learning to Focus your mind, however, isn't always as easy as turning a knob on the TV. For example, have you ever been in class or a meeting and, instead of hearing the speaker, you were preoccupied with wondering what's for lunch. Or, perhaps you've reread the same page of a book over and over, without being able to recall what you just read. We all have times when we are unfocused. However, when we are not focused spiritually, it's like trying to read a book with missing pages.

Sometimes it may feel like your mind is a couch potato surfing from channel to channel at high speed. When you are holding a yoga posture, the unfocused mind will have a field day. It will come up with all sorts of reasons why you should come out of a pose early. It will tell you that you've had enough even when your body can maintain it

longer. It will try to convince you that you should've stayed in bed.

When the mind wanders, gently bring it back as if you were calling a small child to sit beside you. Enlist the powerful guidance of your internal control system to refocus your attention and to recall that your goal is to clear rather than clutter the mind.

Focus requires you to reaffirm your commitment to your bottom-line purpose. This requires practice, clarity, and distinction. In a world where the amount of information we receive doubles each year, the art of discrimination is a necessity. Without Focus, our life is like walking into the New York Public Library and wondering which books are worth reading.

One way to direct the mind is to use a practical tool—one that nearly every meditative tradition offers. It is a technique that protects or guards the mind from intrusive thoughts by using sound repetition. Similar to the rosary beads of Catholicism, Hindu practitioners often use a string of *mala* beads when they chant a *mantra*. Mantra is a sacred thought or prayer repeated over and over again. It consists of Sanskrit words or sentences, many of which are thought to contain healing properties or to bring the

YOGA STORY FOR FOCUS: LESLIE SIMMONS

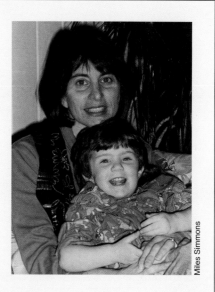

Miles Simmons

When a woman goes into labor, she is charting unknown territory. The unpredictable nature of birth is often very scary. Most of us would prefer not to Focus on pain when we are in the middle of it, yet fighting it can often make it worse. Leslie Simmons intuitively drew upon her knowledge of the Ocean Breath to keep her tuned in and focused on life's greatest miracle—the birth of her first daughter, Liza.

Being in labor is like holding a *really* hard yoga posture. The Ocean Breath was a great gift—without drugs I could not only hold the posture (of labor), but also go deeper into it. I was definitely in pain, but the rhythmic, soothing Ocean Breath was my bridge between the physical intensity and the amazing spiritual experience I was having.

The twelve hours of intense labor were a meditation guided by my use of the Ocean Breath. At first the breath was conscious, but eventually it was completely unconscious and led me into an altered state.

I had never planned to use the Ocean Breath for my whole labor experience, but it was clearly a blessing that I pulled out of my years of yoga practice. It brought the perfect focusing tool together with an ecstatic feeling of union. I imagined myself lying at the water's edge, feeling it wash up (on the inhalation) and down (on the exhalation) into my pelvis.

Other times, the inhalation brought forth the image of a huge owl whose beautiful brown feathers spread wide with each contraction. The soothing exhalations were accompanied by the fiery reds, oranges, and pinks of the sunrise outside my window. I became conscious of my universal connection to every other woman who has ever had a baby or was having one at that same moment. That amazing breath helped me to stay focused and deeply relaxed during my baby's entrance into the world.

---

practitioner into higher states of consciousness.

It is believed that sounds that have been chanted or spoken over thousands of years are imbued with accumulated strength and power. When recited thousands of times over a lifetime, the mantra can be a soothing way to steady the mind during times of crisis and even in the transition to death.

Create your own mantra using one of the twelve Spiritual Muscles, or any other word or words that are meaningful to you. Let the word help you form an intention for your yoga practice. Try to match the words to the rhythm of your breath. Coordinating sound vibration with breath enhances your concentration ability.

During your yoga practice, turn your Focus inward. Practice "spotlighting" in each posture by returning to proper alignment. The more deeply you become absorbed in your experience on the

yoga mat, the deeper you will develop Focus in your daily life. The quality of your yoga experience will depend upon your ability to Focus on such details as specific body parts, movements, form, and breath. When you build the Spiritual Muscle of Focus, you hold postures longer, stronger, and with more integrity. Changing your mind's channel to the subtle nuances of each posture allows you to concentrate on the details of life.

Postures for Focus The Shoulder Opener, Eagle, Chair Pose, Spinal Twist, Half-Boat, and Full Boat sharpens your concentration skills.

Breathing Lesson for Focus The Ocean Breath is designed to engage your Focus in the life-sustaining qualities of breath.

Relaxation for Focus Polarity Relaxation enables you to hone your concentration skills in a deeply soothing manner.

YOGA FOR TWO: SHARING YOGA WITH YOUR UNBORN BABY

As a pregnant woman, you need to nurture yourself (and your baby) more than ever. The dramatic changes you are going through require attention. There will never be another time in your life that you will be more connected to another being. Your body is now the temple for two spirits. Many women have spiritual experiences during pregnancy and labor. Many do not. Allow your pregnancy to be your own unique journey without comparing it to others. Seek the advice and tutelage of a yoga instructor who is certified to teach pregnant woman. Or call 1-800-433-5523 to find a Positive Pregnancy Parenting Fitness instructor in your area. Always consult your health care provider to discuss your individual circumstances. The following do's and don'ts are general safety tips for moms-to-be:

The Don'ts:

1. Never do inverted poses or postures on your belly when you are pregnant or for about two months postpartum. While you should take every opportunity to elevate your feet, raise them only a few inches above your heart. Even extending your legs straight up against a wall (as in the Legs-Up-the-Wall Corpse Pose in the Compassion chapter) is not recommended, as it hinders circulation.

2. Do not lie on your back for long periods of time after the fifth month as it puts pressure on the vena cava. Practice relaxation lying on your left side, which enhances circulation. Use pillows under your belly, between your legs, or wherever you need to.

3. The hormone relaxin, present in the body during pregnancy, may make you more flexible than usual. Do not overstretch during this time. Your body may not be able to return to normal when you are postpartum.

4. Always stop any exercise if you feel strained, overly hot, or tired. Stretch gently and slowly without force. If you tend to get dizzy, don't put your head below your heart—it can cause a head rush or dizziness.

5. Never hold your breath. Don't practice any rapid or forceful breathing during pregnancy. Always allow your breathing to be fluid and steady to keep the oxygen supply available to yourself and your baby.

The Do's:

1. *Listen to your body.* You know your body and its messages better than anyone. Trust your intuitions and trust your body.

2. Do maintain good standing and sitting posture. It may take a little extra effort, but proper alignment will make a world of difference in supporting your changing and growing body. Try squatting as an alternative to always sitting. It will prove valuable throughout your pregnancy and is a wonderful position for birth.

3. Invite your partner to stretch and relax with you. Talk to your baby and practice relaxation techniques so that the whole family feels calm and comfortable.

4. Develop body awareness and practice consciously relaxing various parts of the body on a regular basis. Knowing the difference between tension and relaxation can help you save energy for when you really need it.

5. Develop a support system and a supportive environment for yourself. Work with your fears as they arise. Remember: fear causes tension and tightness in the body. We all have fears, but practicing relaxation techniques and giving yourself plenty of love and care will help you through the exciting journey into motherhood.

SHOULDER OPENER

Body Benefits:

➤ Opens and frees movement in shoulder joints

➤ Helps correct poor posture by aligning spine

➤ Expands chest

➤ Improves respiration

Let's Begin:

1. Come into Proper Standing Alignment. Focus your attention on a point on the wall ahead of you at eye level. Keep your attention at this point for the duration of this posture.

2. Stretch your right arm overhead and extend your left arm down by your side.

3. Bending at the elbow, lower your right hand behind you toward the left shoulder. Then slide it in so that the fingertips point directly down your spine and the elbow points upward.

4. Now draw your left hand up to meet the right by

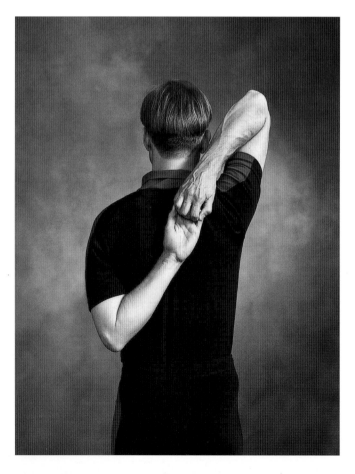

When to avoid this posture Do not practice Shoulder Opener if you have any inflammation or recent injury in the shoulders.

Yoga Tip The shoulders are one of the most telling signs of our emotional states. Some counselors explain that the *should*ers are where we hold our "shoulds." A school of massage therapy called Rolfing claims that the shoulders carry memories of *should*ering heavy burdens and responsibilities. Hike your shoulders up around your ears. What qualities do you sense—fear, insecurity, shock? Hunch your shoulders forward and you'll notice that you feel vulnerable or overwhelmed. Square your shoulders and notice if you feel more proud and self-assured. Return your Focus time and time again to this story-telling part of the body. This warm up will allow the shoulders and your corresponding emotions to feel open and relaxed.

bending it at the elbow and sliding the back side of the hand up your spine.

5. If possible, connect fingertips and draw the right elbow up in a dynamic stretch. If you cannot touch fingertips, simply continue to reach the hands towards each other or clasp your shirt.

6. Breathe deeply and hold this shoulder opening exercise for at least five breaths.

7. To release, *slowly* separate fingertips and extend the arms to their previous positions as in steps 2 and 3. Gently lower the right arm back down to your side.

8. Switch arms and repeat steps 1–7.

9. When you have opened the shoulders on both sides, stand in Proper Standing Alignment with your eyes closed and take several breaths. Notice your attention being drawn into the shoulder area. Take your emotional temperature and compare it to how you felt before you did this exercise.

CHAIR POSE

Body Benefits:

➤ Strengthens joints and leg muscles

➤ Tones abdominal organs

➤ Strengthens back muscles

➤ Helps relieve rheumatism, arthritis, and gout in legs

➤ Stimulates digestion, circulation, and respiration

➤ Builds heat and energy in the body

When to avoid this posture Be gentle and avoid holding for long periods if you have high blood pressure, a history of heart disease, or nervous disorders, or if you are pregnant.

Yoga Tip This pose is so challenging that it will be difficult *not* to Focus on the sensations. The mind loves detail. The Chair Pose invites you into the here and now by encouraging bodily sensations that you can Focus on. The question is: can you achieve *relaxed* Focus? Play with developing a gentle quality to your willful and directed action.

Let's begin:

1. Come into Proper Standing Alignment. Focus your attention on a point on the wall ahead of you, at eye level. Keep your attention at this point for the duration of the posture.

2. Lift your arms straight out in front of you, shoulder distance apart, palms down. Keep the elbows straight and fingertips together. Your arms are parallel to the floor.

3. Imagine that there is a chair behind you. Bend your knees (being careful not to let the knees come together) and lift your hips and buttocks out behind you as if you were trying to sit on the edge of this imaginary seat. Maintain a definite curve in your lower back.

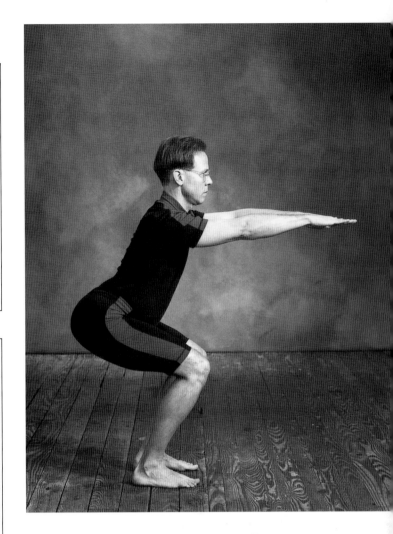

4. Try to move some of the weight onto your heels without losing balance.

5. Come only as far down as feels challenging but not painful.

6. Hold for several breaths, being mindful of your alignment: knees over ankles, head in line with your spine, arms parallel to the floor. Maintain your visual Focus and keep your attention fixed on the details of bodily sensations: heat, tingling, shaking, heaviness, tension, or anything else. Where can you relax while you hold?

7. When you are ready to release, feel your feet rooted in the ground and press down into them to draw your body back up.

8. When you are once again standing, slowly release your arms back down to your sides.

9. Close your eyes and allow your breath to return to normal. Tune into the sensations as they change.

EAGLE

Body Benefits:

➤ Improves digestion and relieves constipation

➤ Strengthens and flexes all major joints

➤ Loosens and opens shoulders

➤ Removes and prevents leg cramps

➤ Supplies fresh blood to kidneys and reproductive organs

➤ Tones legs, abdomen, and upper arms

When to avoid this posture Be gentle and avoid holding it for long periods if you have high blood pressure, a history of heart disease, or nervous disorders, or if you are pregnant.

Yoga Tip The eagle is known as the king of birds. In Native American tradition, it is honored as the ultimate seer of things in the animal kingdom. Unlike the eagle, which uses its naked eye, when *you* want to see an object that is small or far away, you use a magnifying glass. This makes even tiny particles look bigger and more significant. This pose is like a giant magnifying glass. It encourages you to Focus on every part of your body. Even your fingers and toes are engaged and focused to create the form of the Eagle. Remember: fixing the eyes on one point on the wall will encourage the development of Focus.

Let's begin:

1. Come into Proper Standing Alignment but with your feet and legs pressed together tightly. Focus your attention on a point on the wall ahead of you at eye level. Keep your attention at this point for the duration of the posture.

2. Bend your knees and lower your body several inches, keeping your spine straight.

3. Draw your arms out to the side and then cross

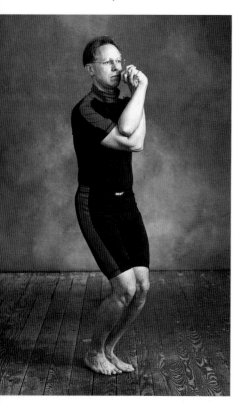

them in front of you with the left arm on top of the right. Bend the elbows and bring your forearms up toward your face. If possible, clasp hands and interlace the fingers, or simply press the arms together as if you were trying to keep any air from moving between them.

4. BREATHE!!! It is easy to forget to breathe when you are in deep concentration.

5. This may be as far as you can go at first. When you are ready to engage the legs, move on to step 6.

6. Imagine that you are sitting in a chair and want to cross your legs. Keeping the left leg bent and steady, lift the right leg up and cross it over the left. If possible, tuck the toes of the right leg around the left ankle. Focus on pressing the legs together tightly.

7. Hold this balancing and focusing posture for five to ten breaths or as long as you can. Concentrate on your visual spot and on pressing the arms and legs together.

8. To release, unwrap the right leg from the left and place it back down beside the bent left leg. Straighten the legs and then unravel the arms, spreading them out to either side like eagle wings and then back down by your sides.

9. Stand with the eyes closed and check in.

10. Repeat the Eagle with the opposite side, replacing "left" for "right" on steps 1–9.

11. Once you have completed both sides, remain in Proper Standing Alignment with your eyes closed and check in with yourself.

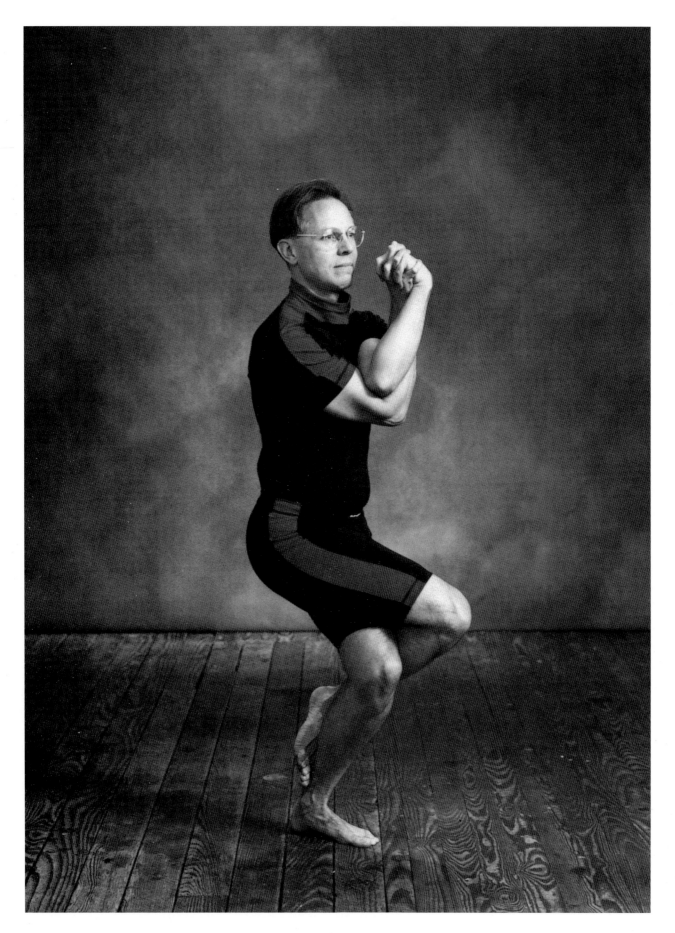

SPINAL TWIST

Body Benefits:

➤ Rotates, flexes, extends, and aligns spine

➤ Tones abdominals

➤ Stimulates liver and spleen

➤ Increases flexibility in hips

➤ Activates peristalsis (digestion)

➤ Relieves constipation

➤ Reduces stiffness in shoulders and neck

➤ Increases circulation

➤ Brings fresh oxygen to musculoskeletal system

When to avoid this posture If you have had abdominal hernia, do not practice the Spinal Twist.

Yoga Tip Draw your Focus to the spine. Notice how it is the core of your being. See your other body parts in relation to this dynamic center. As your spine lengthens, what happens to the breath? As the spine twists, what other parts of the body are affected? The thirty-two bones of the spinal column (or vertebrae) form within the first month of pregnancy. The Spinal Twist is a wonderful way to pay homage to this supple and significant part of your body.

Let's begin:

1. Sit on your buttocks with your legs stretched out in front of you. Feel your sitting bones, the two knobs at the base of your pelvis, in contact with the ground.

2. Bend the right leg at the knee and draw it up toward your chest. Place the right foot flat on the floor next to the left knee, or (for greater challenge) cross it over onto the left side of the left knee.

3. The left leg remains straight throughout this part of the posture. Flex the toes back toward your face and push the left heel away from your body.

4. Place your left hand on your right knee, or wrap the left elbow around that bent knee.

5. Stretch out the right arm directly in front of you. Swing the right hand around the body to the right until it is behind you. Your eyes should follow your right hand, creating a twist to the spine.

6. Place the right palm down on the ground, close to the spine to keep yourself upright. Press the palm into the ground with the fingertips pointing away from you.

7. Each time you inhale, lengthen the spine as if you were growing taller. With each exhalation, twist the spine just a hair more as you look over the right shoulder.

8. As a beginner, take three to five breaths in this posture. With practice, you will be able to hold it longer.

9. Relax your facial muscles and any others that don't need to be working in this posture.

10. To release, lift the right hand off the floor and begin to slowly circle it back in front of you. Let the right arm come down to rest at your side.

11. As if you are in meditation, slowly change your leg position. The right leg is now outstretched on the ground, and the left knee is bent up toward the chest.

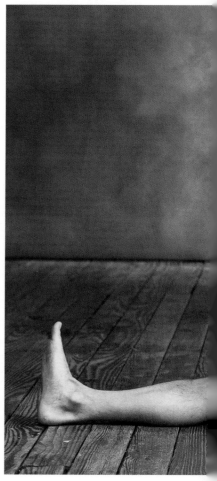

12. Repeat the Spinal Twist to the left, following steps 2–10.

13. When you have completed both sides, sit in a comfortable position with eyes closed and check in to notice how you are feeling.

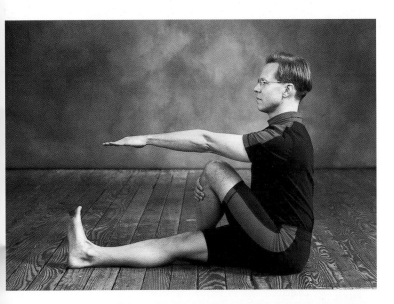

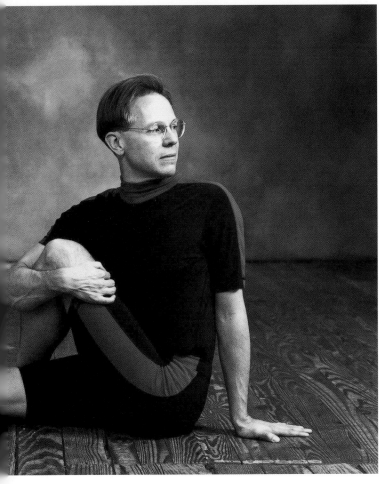

CREATE YOUR OWN POSTURE FOR FOCUS

Let's begin:

1. Practice the formal yoga postures before you begin. Come into a comfortable seated position with your eyes closed.

2. Connect deeply with your breath, becoming absorbed in its flow in and out of your body. The Focus of this experience is to bring the breath deeply into the body.

3. In slow motion, begin to stretch in ways that open up your breathing even deeper. Reach to the left, press your rib cage around in circles, and open the neck area.

4. Continuously find ways to expand your breathing capacity through slow, expansive movement. Remain inwardly focused, following the movement of your breath as if you were a private investigator.

5. Try to involve every possible part of your body. Keep the Focus on how your movements allow the breath to flow more easily.

6. When you find a posture that feels particularly intriguing or that you wish to explore in minute detail and through micro-movements, stay there.

7. Notice the texture of the posture, its subtle nuances, shape, and energy.

8. Stay in this position for several breaths. Open your eyes if you wish.

9. Make a note of the posture you have created. You may want to draw a picture of it or write about it. Create an affirmation about how you want Focus to be a part of your life, and repeat it when you are in this posture. Give it a name and add it to your Focus repertoire or create a new posture each time.

HALF-BOAT

Body Benefits:

➤ Strengthens and tones back, thighs, and arm muscles

➤ Oxygenates kidneys

➤ Revitalizes entire system

➤ Helps maintain bladder and prostate gland

➤ Stimulates functions of internal organs

➤ Stretches front of body

➤ Expands chest and strengthens lungs

➤ Strengthens digestive and reproductive systems

➤ Assists relief of menstrual discomforts

When to avoid this posture Do not practice Half-Boat or Boat if you have had recent abdominal surgery or inflammation, hernia, hypertension, or if you are pregnant or menstruating.

Yoga Tip In any posture where you are lying belly down, you will press into the pelvic triangle. The pelvic triangle is formed by the two hip bones and the pubic bone. As you lie on your belly, squeeze the buttocks and simultaneously press the pelvic triangle into the floor. This is your anchor for the Boat posture. (Get it? Anchor . . . boat? OK, you get the picture.)

Let's begin:

1. Lie on your belly, legs together. Extend your feet away from your head. Squeeze the buttocks and press the pelvic triangle down into the floor. Wiggle your torso out of your waist as though you are an inchworm. Relax the shoulders and press the crown of your head away from the feet.

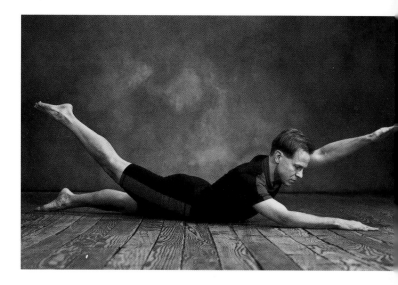

2. Stretch your arms out in front of you on the ground.

3. Stretch the *right* arm (palm down) and the *left* leg (toes pointed) away from each other. Then lift them off the ground along with the head and shoulders. Keep your head in line with your spine, gazing down in front of your grounded hand. Keep your Focus at this point for the duration of this posture.

4. Breathe steadily and hold for three to five breaths or longer, if you can. Notice what it feels like to stretch and elongate the body.

5. Keep the buttocks squeezed as you slowly lower the right arm and left leg.

6. Now, lift the *left* arm and the *right* leg away from each other and off the ground along with the head and shoulders. Take three to five breaths in this position.

7. Keep the buttocks squeezed as you lower the left arm and the right leg back to the floor.

8. Release the squeeze in the buttocks, turn your head to one side, and take a moment to relax completely.

9. You may wish to transition slowly in the Child Pose before you enter the full Boat posture.

The one sustenance, the great sustaining power all mankind can receive, is strength from God. If you are sick in body, weary in mind, despondent and hopeless, turn your thoughts away from yourself. Turn your thoughts and your prayers and your praise to God; focus your whole heart and mind upon God. Never waver, never falter, hold fast to belief in the Great White Spirit; and in God's light you will find that every need of your life will be met.

— WHITE EAGLE

BOAT

The benefits and contraindications of the Boat are the same as for the Half-Boat.

> *Yoga Tip* This is a challenging posture. Imagine that you are a strong, stable boat. Your boat, or body, will rock steadily with the movement of your breath. Remember to keep your breath fluid and moving. Use the breath to help you remain focused, energized, and conscious.

Let's begin:

1. Begin on the floor, on your belly. Your arms are extended in front of you. Your legs are as close to each other as possible and your forehead rests on the ground.

2. Go through the steps for Proper Standing Alignment even though you are on your belly. Remember to press the pelvic triangle into the floor as you squeeze the buttocks.

3. On an exhalation, lift *both* arms and *both* legs off the ground a few inches or more. Lift the head and shoulders as well.

Reach your hands forward, fingers together, palms facing each other.

4. Breathe! Keep your arms and legs raised for as many breaths as you can without strain. For beginners, start with three.

5. Keep your buttocks squeezed as you lower the body back down to the ground in a slow, controlled release.

6. When your body is back on the ground, release the squeeze in the buttocks. Turn the head to one side and relax completely. Let your body melt into the ground.

7. To relieve any residual tension in the lower back, bend your knees and windshield wipe the lower legs back and forth.

8. Close your eyes and become aware of how your energy has shifted.

9. You may wish to transition slowly in the Child Pose before you create your own posture.

The more deeply I breathe, the more relaxed and focused I am.

— MARIA RODRIGUEZ, YOGA STUDENT

OCEAN BREATH

Body Benefits:

➤ Removes phlegm from throat

➤ Removes impurities from lungs

➤ Calms nerves and absorbs mind in meditative sound

➤ Increases endurance and builds stamina

➤ Can be practiced throughout entire yoga session

➤ Helps use entire lung capacity and aerates lungs

➤ Increases body heat, which aids flexibility

➤ Improves some respiratory (including asthma) and circulatory ailments

➤ Is safe for most anyone

Yoga Tip I have nicknamed this the Darth Vader Breath because of the rhythmic sound it creates. You are already familiar with the Ocean Breath, as it is the technique used when you whisper. It is easiest to learn this breathing technique with your mouth open. Once you have mastered it, you can perform it with a closed mouth. Your mind will become entranced with its soothing, rhythmic, uniform sound. Many people use this breath to help alleviate cravings and addictions. I had a twenty-four-year-old female student who smoked two packs of cigarettes a day for eight years. She uses the Ocean Breath as a replacement for a drag on a cigarette. The Ocean Breath washed away her addiction, and she has been smoke-free for more than four years! The Sanskrit name for this technique, *ujjai,* literally means "that which leads to victory." Allow this breath to lead you to triumph.

Let's begin:

1. Come into Proper Sitting Alignment with your eyes closed.

2. Imagine that you have a mirror in front of you. Hold your hand out in front of you to represent this imaginary mirror.

3. Inhale through your nose. As you exhale, imagine that you are fogging the mirror whispering, "Aaah."

4. Repeat this several times, becoming absorbed in the sound you are making. You can lower your hand into your lap at this point and close your lips.

5. With mouth closed, imagine a mirror at the back of your throat. As you inhale, try to fog this mirror as well directing the "Aaah" sound to the back of your throat with a closed mouth. You will feel a slight constriction in your throat.

6. Exhale with the mouth still closed, try to fog the imaginary mirror in front of you as you did with the mouth open.

7. Repeat steps 5 and 6 for ten to twenty breaths. Stop at any point if you feel lightheaded or are straining.

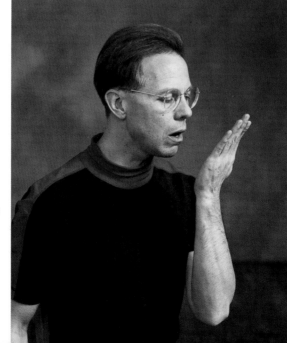

8. Become absorbed in the sound you are creating. The sound resembles the ebb and flow of the ocean tide. Allow your breath to wash over you like gentle waves on a pleasant beach.

9. When you are finished, allow your breath to go back to its normal rhythm and notice the effect on your body and mind.

POLARITY RELAXATION

Let's begin:

1. Assume the Corpse Pose. Take several full, deep, long breaths.

2. Imagine that your body is inside a large, safe bubble. Become fascinated by the movement of your breath within your body. Imagine that your breath is like a magical wave that can come in and out like the tide in whatever way you direct it.

3. As you inhale, allow the movement of your breath to come in through the soles of your feet and travel in a straight path up the legs, through the pelvis and the torso, and out through the top of your head. On the exhalation, it passes out through the top of the head. Imagine that you have a whale's blowhole at the crown of your head. Repeat this sequence for the next ten breaths.

4. Now reverse the direction. As you inhale, draw the breath through the crown of your head down through the torso and pelvis, then the legs, and out through the soles of your feet. Feel the wave of your breath as it travels naturally in this direction. Relax into the breathing. Continue for ten breaths.

5. Now imagine that you can draw your breath in through the left palm, up the arm, and across the chest. Exhale the breath down the right arm through the right palm. Let your breath flow naturally like a wave across the body. Notice how effortless it is to do this.

6. Now reverse the direction and let the breath wave come through the right palm and across the body. Exhale it through the left palm. Repeat for ten breaths.

7. Next draw the air in through the sole of the left foot, up the leg, and into the pelvis. Exhale air down the right leg and out the sole of the right foot. Repeat for ten breaths.

8. Switch sides. Inhale through the sole of the right foot, into the pelvis, and out through the sole of the left foot. Repeat for ten breaths.

9. Imagine that your body is divided into halves—the back half that is in contact with the ground and the front half that faces upward. Bring the breath into the body from the entire back half and let it wash out through the front. Let go of the sense that you are directing this at all and simply watch it happen for ten more breaths.

10. Absorb the inhalation through the front side of your body now, and let it go through the back into the ground below. Do this ten more times. Feel your body melt into the floor.

11. Imagine someone with a giant paintbrush who can paint the movement of your breath up and down your spine. Allow the paintbrush to move up the length of your spine from tailbone to cervical vertebrae, then back down. Sense the fluidity and ease of movement of the breath through your body. Repeat ten times more.

12. Finally, let the breath travel everywhere, in every direction, delivering fresh oxygen to each and every cell. Sense the movement as a brilliant and graceful dance. Observe this flow for a few minutes.

13. When you feel complete, deepen your breath and begin to slowly wiggle the fingertips and toes. As you are ready, gradually roll over to one side, hugging your knees to your chest.

14. Come up slowly and sit for a few moments with your eyes closed. Attune to the sensations you feel.

Yoga has improved my concentration by teaching me to focus on one task at a time.

—EUCARIS MONTANEZ, YOGA STUDENT

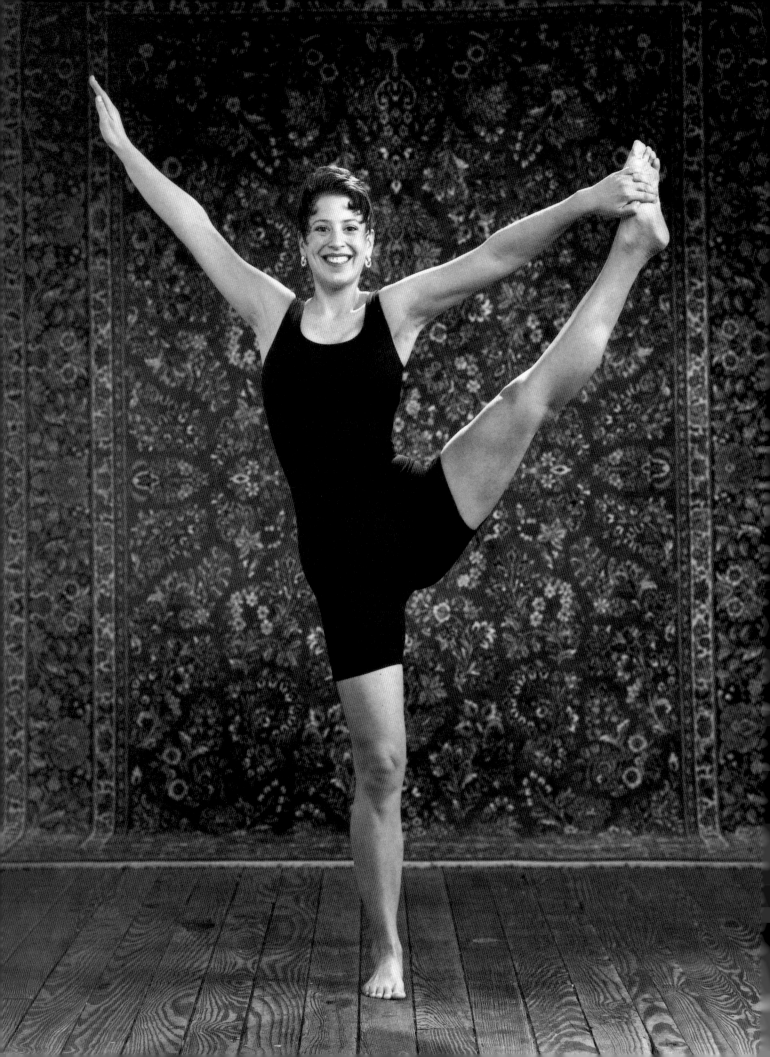

FLEXIBILITY

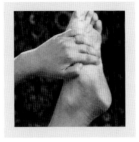

Imagine your body and mind as a magical boat that travels to exotic lands. To fully explore these unusual places, meet interesting people, and gain new perspectives, you need to drop anchor for awhile. However, if you leave the anchor down permanently in some safe harbor, you close yourself off to other experiences. You become stuck, able to see things only from a single vantage point. While being anchored to one spot provides a sense of safety, it can also be constricting and isolating. Developing the Spiritual Muscle of Flexibility allows you to weigh anchor and explore alternative ways of seeing and being. To be flexible is to be free.

When you were a baby, you were incredibly flexible, so much so that you could touch your feet to your head. If you tried that now, you might be screaming rather than cooing. Babies are naturally flexible. They are free from tensions and stress that can cause rigidity and stiffness. We all have the potential to return to a more pliable state of being.

By the same token, as a small child, you fantasized, dreamed, and imagined. Nothing, not even the way you ate your food, had specific or strict rules. (Perhaps you were one of those who created highways and roads in your mashed potato mountains.) Certainly, as an adult you need to develop habits that help structure your life, but bodies and minds function better when they are flexible.

Rigidly clinging to outworn beliefs, desires, and especially fears can contribute to dis-ease. When we are inflexible, it is as though we are in a fight with our own bodies and minds. What if a tree were as inflexible as our minds can be? Any storm that passed through could cause the tree to snap—even tear it from the earth by its roots. Luckily, trees sway and adapt to most weather conditions. You can train your mind to do the same.

Native peoples are flexible in their thinking, their attitudes, and their bodies. They open themselves to the spirit world often through music and dance. One of the oldest cultures in West Africa, the Yoruba, enjoys numerous celebrations featuring drummers and dancers. A Yoruba dancer must respond spontaneously to the rhythms of the

Be as still as a mountain, move like a great river.

—FROM THE ESSENCE OF T'AI CHI CH'UAN, TRANSLATED AND EDITED BY
BENJAMIN PANG JENG LO

drums, just as the soul of each observer must be open to messages from the gods.

Some aboriginal tribes assert that we are all related to animals, and they see in animal behavior metaphors for their own lives. In Marlo Morgan's *Mutant Message Down Under*, she notes:

> *The slithering snake is a learning tool when we observe its frequent removal of the outer skin. Little is gained in a lifetime if what you believe at age seven is still how you feel at age thirty-seven. It is necessary to shed old ideas, habits, opinions, and even companions sometimes. Letting go is sometimes a very difficult human lesson. The snake is no lesser nor greater for shedding the old. It is just necessary.*

Another powerful example of aboriginal Flexibility involves names. Although every child is named at birth, each person chooses another name at adulthood. The new name represents that person's current role in society. It is hoped that individuals will have many names throughout their lives, as this symbolizes a life redefined with clear purpose.

Flexibility, or flowing with change, is a life skill. How often do you have to adjust and compromise in your relationships with your family, fellow workers, or even other drivers on the street? When we are willing to accept life only as we want it to be,

we lack spontaneity, vigor, humor, and dexterity. The cultivation of Flexibility permits us to bend in the storms that inevitably touch all human lives and to emerge into the calm that follows with our spirits intact.

Instead of worrying about how to perform the yoga steps perfectly, let your body find its own rhythm, its own truth for each posture. That is the beauty of flexibility! Adapt the movements to fit your current state of wellness. Keep your body safe by keeping it warm—even iron will yield when it's hot. Let the bends and rotations serve as a soothing salve to the joints and systems of your body. Bask in the luxurious stretches and twists that yoga teaches.

Postures for Flexibility All of the yoga postures featured in this book help you become more limber. When practiced as a series, the Wrist Pulls, Palm Presses, Straddle-Fold Twist, Sun Prayer, and Knee-Down Twist flex every major muscle of the body. You can also be flexible when creating your own posture. Remember, you are limited only by your imagination.

Breathing Lesson for Flexibility The Three-Part Breath encourages mobility in the chest. It invites you to use all of your breathing apparatus rather than just a small portion of it.

Visualization for Flexibility Anchors Aweigh! takes you on an imaginative journey to discover new ways of thinking about current situations.

Spiritual maturity allows us, like bamboo, to move in the wind, to respond to the world with our under-standing and our hearts, to respect the changing circumstances around us. The spiritually mature person has learned the great arts of staying present and letting go. Their flexibility understands that there is not just one way of practice or one fine spiritual tradition, but there are many ways. It understands that spiritual life is not about adopting any one particular philosophy or set of beliefs or teachings, that it is not a cause for taking a stand in opposition to someone else or something else. It is an easiness of heart that understands that all of the spiritual vehicles are rafts to cross the stream to freedom.

—FROM A PATH WITH HEART, BY JACK KORNFIELD

YOGA STORY FOR FLEXIBILITY: MORRIS RUBIN

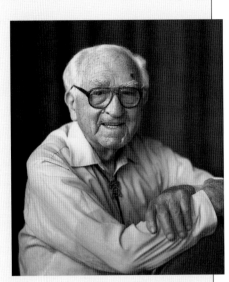

Morris Rubin, born in Russia on November 15, 1900 (ninety-six years young at the time of our interview), is not your typical retired lawyer. First of all, he has outlived most of his colleagues. He also practices yoga every day and gives yoga demonstrations. He calls himself "Morris 'Available' Rubin, one-man social service agency." He has more agility than many of my college-age students. He credits yoga for his remarkable Flexibility—and the fact that he hasn't had so much as a headache or sore throat since he began practicing.

When I was sixty-four years old, I felt a little run down. I was going from doctor to doctor with no results. Nothing was wrong with me, but I felt lousy. My wife, May, and I found a yoga class, and I've been in the yoga business ever since.

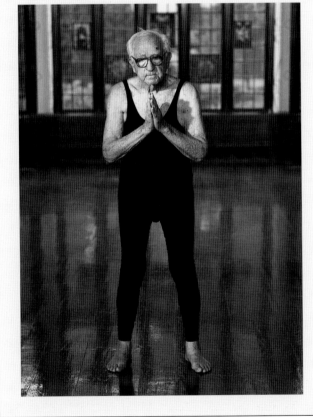

Because of an old football injury to my spine, I have some trouble jumping around. If I didn't do yoga, I'd probably be in a wheelchair by now. I practice yoga religiously. By that I don't mean with a Bible in my hand, but rather seven days a week (no vacations).

Motion is everything. My advice is to continue to move as long as you can. Whatever you can move, *move!* I have no arthritis; in fact, I haven't got a pain in my body. Every part of my body receives attention in yoga. Many of the postures I designed myself to suit my own needs. I call them "yoga for Morris Rubin." You have to respect your body and its capabilities.

Yoga prepares me for the day. When I'm practicing, I'm not thinking about anything else. I'm just doing yoga. Afterward, I take the benefits from yoga and help other people. I take a few older women who live alone to do their shopping, and then I help them unload the groceries. Yoga undoubtedly makes me a better person.

When people are born they are supple, and when they die they are stiff. When trees are born they are tender, and when they die they are brittle. Stiffness is thus a companion of death, flexibility a companion of life. So when an army is strong, it does not prevail. When a tree is strong, it is cut for use. So the stiff and strong are below, the supple and yielding on top.

—FROM THE ESSENTIAL TAO, *TRANSLATED AND PRESENTED BY THOMAS CLEARY*

IT'S NEVER TOO LATE: YOGA INTO YOUR 100S

Our society is obsessed with looking and staying young. A lot of time, money, and energy are spent in the attempt to mask aging. Luckily, people like Ram Dass and Rabbi Zalman Schachter are bringing profound consciousness to this natural process. Rabbi Schacter is the founder of The Spiritual Eldering Institute and, along with Ron Miller, wrote the book and coined the refreshing phrase, *From Age-ing to Sage-ing.*™

Yoga respects the aging process and, without doubt, helps us to *feel* young. One of the main reasons I love yoga is that it's a satisfying resource that we can use throughout our whole lives. It is extremely versatile and easily adapted—a genuine lifestyle habit. In addition, the benefits are so far reaching that they encompass the entire gamut of life situations. Do you know the saying, "If you can walk, you can dance?" Well, how about this adaptation: "If you're alive, you can do yoga." When you are in your sage-ing years, consider the following:

1. Allow yourself to be surprised. In one Elderhostel course, the most common expression I heard was, "Wow, I didn't think my body could do this!" Imagine you are an explorer seeking out new adventures with your body.

2. Adapt postures to meet your current needs. For example, instead of practicing Straddle-Fold Twist the way it is shown in this chapter, try it while sitting in a chair. Bring your torso forward and touch your left toes with your right hand. Reach the left hand overhead. You'll get the same twisting benefit and open up more possibilities for yourself.

3. By the same token, you don't have to stand for most of the traditional standing poses. Standing for long periods of time is strenuous. Try a seated Mountain and a seated Half-Moon. Speaking of chairs, don't be afraid to use them as props to help maintain balance. I often use a chair or a wall to help build confidence and for safety.

4. Move slowly to gradually develop greater elasticity. One of the most noticeable losses when we don't move regularly is range of motion—in hips, shoulders, torso, and every other part of the body. Yoga increases your range of mobility.

5. Practice the breathing techniques often. The breath has been a constant companion since the day you were born. It can help reduce irritability, increase vitality, and calm the nerves.

6. Don't isolate yourself! Invite people to join you. One winter, my husband and I were visiting his parents in Florida. They are really fun people and we decided to do yoga outside on the beach. Not only did we enjoy ourselves, but other people in their condominium asked to join us.

Thanks to yoga, I feel like I can move in any direction like an elastic band.

—JEANINE HOMELAND, YOGA STUDENT

7. Keep moving! Part of what slows us down as we age is inactivity itself. The yoga postures are designed to stimulate the functioning of all physiological systems. Virtually every part of your body and mind works more effectively with regular yoga practice.

8. While our culture does not encourage us to let out sound, yoga definitely does. During some of the postures, you might feel like sighing, letting out an "Mmmm" or other noises. One Elderhostel student told me she left yoga feeling great, even better than after her Thursday lunches with her girlfriends. "I felt like someone really listened to me—I did!"

9. Create a healthy framework for your day by designating a specific time for yoga. While we all enjoy free time, most of my senior friends tell me that the hardest part of retirement is the lack of structure. Establish a ritual to mark the beginning and end of your yoga practice.

10. Teach others. Share your good fortune with friends, family, or coworkers. Erase age stereotypes and become a role model for younger people.

11. If you are new to yoga, trust that you are on a fabulous inner and outer journey. Be patient and enjoy the ride. As playwright-director Jerome Lawrence (my favorite of his was *Auntie Mame*) said in *The Courage to Grow Old*, "I have always preferred not merely the Pursuit of Happiness, but the Happiness of Pursuit."

12. Maintain a sense of humor. At ninety-three, George Burns made a movie about how he lived his daily life. His mornings consisted of walking many laps around his large outdoor swimming pool, doing his own series of yogalike stretches, and cracking jokes the whole way through.

13. If you don't have a Morris Rubin (this chapter's Yoga Story) as a role model, find one. Check out my favorite books of photography, *Growing Old Is Not for Sissies: Portraits of Senior Athletes* (Volumes I and II) by Etta Clark and Richard Selzer. These remarkable accounts of older athletes in every activity imaginable will surely inspire you.

14. Memory is a precious commodity. When you allow blood to flow to your head, you give your brain a memory treat. You can do this sitting in a chair, as long as you don't have any physical contraindications. Sit at the edge of your chair with your hands on your knees. Drop your chin toward your chest and lean your torso forward as far as is comfortable.

15. Sadie and Bessie Delany, authors of *Having Our Say: The Delany Sisters' First Hundred Years*, stretched for one hour a day with postures as challenging as the Half-Shoulderstand. Even ten minutes a day is beneficial. Eventually, you can increase the time for even greater benefits. Movement is the elixir of life.

The less I criticize myself, the less tense my body becomes.

—JENNIFER BELIKOFF, YOGA STUDENT (AND SOON-TO-BE-YOGA TEACHER)

WRIST PULLS AND PALM PRESSES

Body Benefits:

- ➤ Stretches and contracts side muscles
- ➤ Improves spinal flexibility
- ➤ Regulates kidney functioning
- ➤ Tones and strengthens intercostal, lateral, and dorsal muscles
- ➤ Improves digestion
- ➤ Aids respiration
- ➤ Brings heat and energy to body

Yoga Tip Every part of your body delights in having the room to breathe and move freely without constraint. Eyeballs roll, hearts pump, lungs expand and contract, blood flows, joints rotate, and hair grows. Even your stomach lining renews itself every three days. Try to think of a part of your body that doesn't move, change, or grow in some way. Simply by doing this, your brain generates electrical impulses. If any part of your body is constricted or blocked, it usually indicates *dis*-ease. Your emotions and energy also require space. Give yourself room to have the whole gamut of feelings that a human being can experience in a lifetime.

Let's begin:

1. Come into Proper Standing Alignment with your arms at your sides and your feet hip width apart.

2. Reach both arms overhead. Grab the right wrist with your left hand and pull it up and over to the left. You will feel a stretch from your right hand all the way to the right hip.

3. Take a few deep breaths while stretching out the right side.

4. Bring your arms back directly overhead. Let go of the right wrist.

5. Interlace the fingers and turn your palms up toward the ceiling.

6. Take a few deep breaths while you actively press your palms upward.

7. Release your hands but keep them overhead. Grab the left wrist with your right hand and pull it up and over to the right. This stretch extends from your left hand all the way to the left hip.

8. Take a few deep breaths while stretching the left side of the body.

9. Let go of the left wrist. Slowly relax both arms down to your sides.

10. Where does your body feel more open and spacious? Take a moment to close your eyes and notice any shifts that may have taken place.

These forms are not the means of obtaining the right state of mind. To take this posture is itself to have the right state of mind. There is no need to obtain some special state of mind.

—FROM *ZEN MIND, BEGINNER'S MIND*, BY SHUNRYU SUZUKI

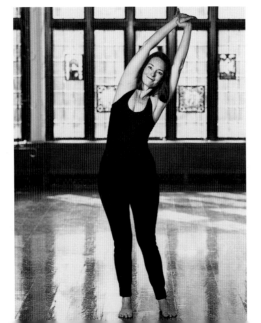

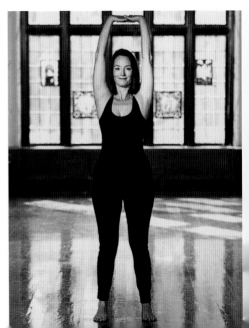

STRADDLE-FOLD TWIST

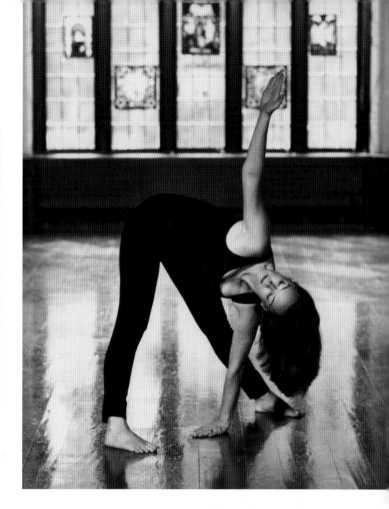

Body Benefits:

➤ Rotates, extends, and aligns spine

➤ Brings fresh supply of blood and oxygen to spine

➤ Stimulates spinal nerves

➤ Activates digestion

➤ Improves hip and neck flexibility

➤ Strengthens muscles of legs, abdomen, and arms

➤ Improves circulation and respiration

Let's begin:

1. Come into Proper Standing Alignment. Inhale a full deep breath.

2. As you exhale, move your feet apart about a leg's length (or three feet).

3. Bend the knees and place your hands just above the knees. Hinge at the hips, straighten the legs, and with a flat back come forward until your torso is parallel to the ground.

4. Place your right hand on the ground between your two feet with the fingers pointing at the left foot. Keep your spine extended, bending the knees if necessary.

5. Draw the left arm overhead until it is parallel to the right arm.

6. Turn to face the raised left hand. If you feel any strain in the neck area, simply look forward, or down toward your right hand.

7. Maintain a lengthened spine even as you twist. Keep breathing into this delicious stretch for five to ten breaths.

8. Lower the left hand until it replaces the right, fingers pointing toward the right foot. Continue on this side from step 5.

9. To release, lower both arms down in front of the body. Walk the feet closer together in a heel-toe-

heel-toe manner. Place your hands on your bent knees, and tuck in the tailbone slightly. Roll up the spine, stacking one vertebra on top of another.

10. Stand with the eyes closed and check in with yourself. Notice the parts of the body that feel more agile.

When to avoid this posture Do not practice Straddle-Fold Twist if you are pregnant.

Yoga Tip When you are truly flexible, you can step out of your traditional way of doing things. Did you know that hummingbirds can fly backwards? The loon can not only fly but also swim underwater and dive to depths of 180 feet. Some fish can actually leap up to forty feet out of the water to avoid attack. Have you ever skipped to find your car in the parking lot? Try picking up your watch with your foot rather than your hand. To be flexible in your movements is to enjoy unique ways of experiencing life.

SUN PRAYER

Body Benefits:

➤ Stretches and strengthens entire system

➤ Invigorates whole body

➤ Limbers spine and joints

➤ Stimulates digestion, elimination, and circulation

➤ Provides fresh oxygen to heart and lungs

➤ Alleviates constipation

➤ Stimulates endocrine glands

➤ Helps develop coordination and poise

➤ Normalizes breathing

➤ Balances nervous system

➤ Helps to correct menstrual irregularity

When to avoid this series If you have uncontrolled high blood pressure, hernia, or venous blood clots, do not perform the Sun Prayer.

Yoga Tip The Sun Prayer is a series of postures that flow together in a beautiful and graceful sequence. It may seem difficult at first, but with practice it will become easier. You'll have it memorized in no time!

Feel free to adapt any of the postures to meet the needs and current limitations of your body.

Make it fun for yourself. Imagine that you are outside at sunrise and offering a prayer of gratitude to the sun. Throughout history, people have honored the sun. Helios was the sun god in Greek myth, while the Egyptian equivalent was called Ra. Some Plains Indians worship the sun in a religious dance at the summer solstice. The first day of the week, Sunday, literally means "day of the sun." Recall the significant role the sun plays in your life and in the lives of all living beings.

Let's begin:

1. Start in Proper Standing Alignment.

2. Use the Natural Breath or the Ocean Breath while performing the Sun Series.

3. Bring your palms together in front of your heart in prayer position. Inhale and lift the arms up overhead with palms together.

4. Squeeze your buttocks and arch back slightly, lifting the chin and chest upward.

5. Separate the palms and hinge at the hips, lowering the torso to a flat-back position (called the Jackknife) with your arms outstretched alongside your head.

6. Release from the Jackknife and hang all the way down in the Rag Doll, head heavy, arms hanging separately.

7. Bend the knees, place both hands on the floor on either side of your feet, and step the right leg back into the Runner's Stretch. Your left knee is bent directly over the left ankle. (If the knee is too far in front of the ankle, you can strain it.)

8. Bring the left leg back to meet the right leg. Your body should look like you are about to do a push-up. The body is in one plane with neck and head in line with the spine.

9. Gently lower both knees to the ground and bring the hips back to rest on the heels. Lower your forehead on or close to the ground with your arms outstretched in front of you in the Child Pose.

10. Pushing with your hips, lift your buttocks, bend the elbows, and bring the nose down toward the ground as if you were looking for a lost contact lens.

11. Slide your head (with your nose close to the floor) and chest past your hands, scooping your torso through the hands.

Watch out, Rolaids! I've found another way to spell relief: Y-O-G-A!

— H O P E   F O L E Y ,   Y O G A   S T U D E N T

---

*When my body is stretching out into the postures,
I feel like my mind is stretching out, too.*

—ILISSA KIRSCHBAUM,
YOGA STUDENT

12. Straighten the legs and balance on your hands and toes (and knees if necessary) in the Up-Facing Dog.

13. Lift the face and look up toward the sun.

14. Press the hips up into the air, pushing with your arms until your body forms a triangle (with the hands, feet, and buttocks). This position is called the Down-Facing Dog.

15. In the Down-facing Dog, your heels reach toward the ground. They may not yet touch the ground. You will feel a pronounced stretch in the backs of the legs.

16. Step the right foot forward, entering the Runner's Stretch on the opposite side.

17. Check to see that the right knee is directly over the right ankle, rather than hyperextended.

18. Lift the hips as you bring the left foot forward to meet the right foot. Hang in the Rag Doll for a moment.

19. If your back is weak, leave the arms hanging as you roll up the spine, stacking the vertebrae. If your back is in good condition, extend your arms alongside your head and lift the torso up with a flat back through the Jackknife position.

20. Once you are standing upright, bring your palms together in prayer position and lift the arms up overhead.

21. Squeeze your buttocks and arch back slightly, lifting the chin and chest toward the ceiling.

22. Return to Proper Standing Alignment and lower the arms back down into prayer position in front of your heart.

23. Take a moment to stand with your eyes closed and feel the effects of this series. You may choose to repeat it to increase your Flexibility.

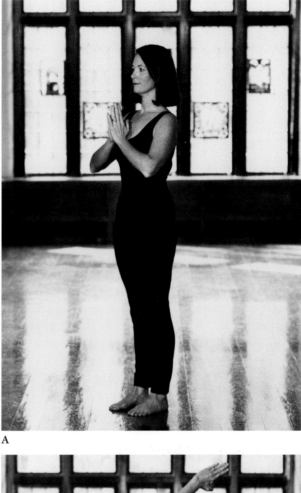

A

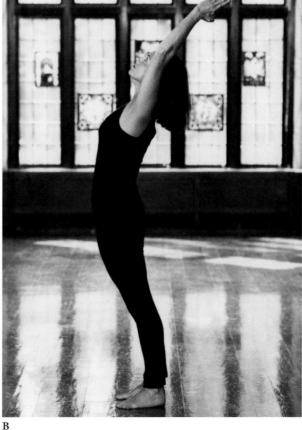

B

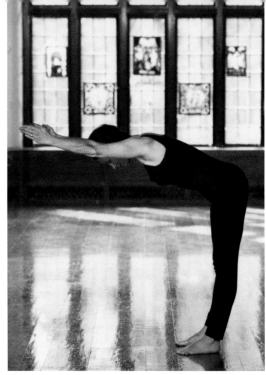

C

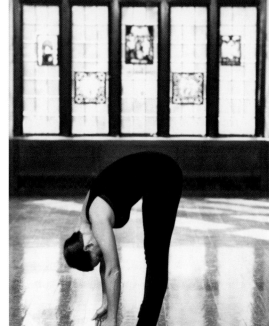

D

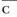E

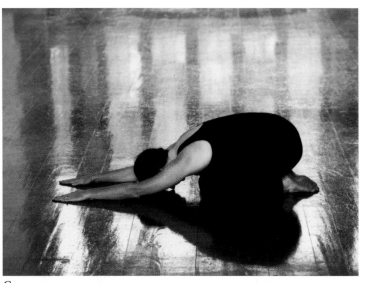

G

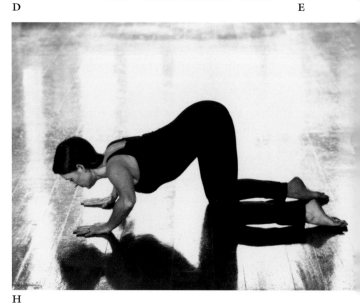

H L

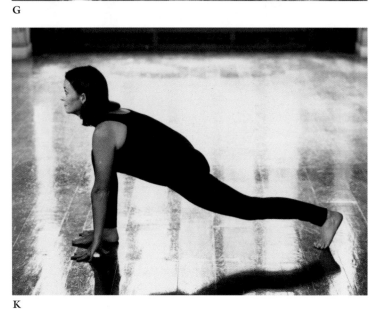

K

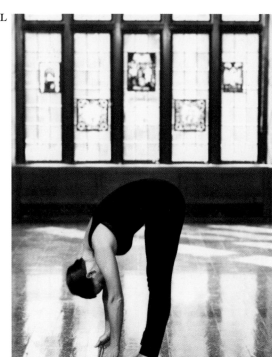

M

66

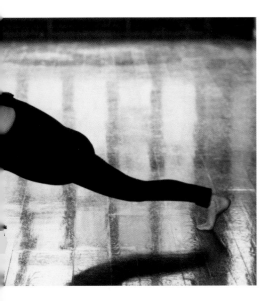

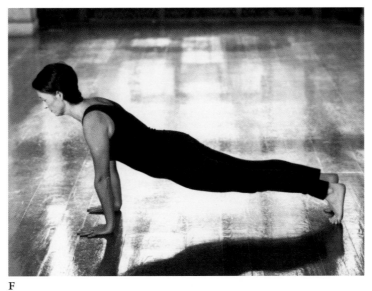

F

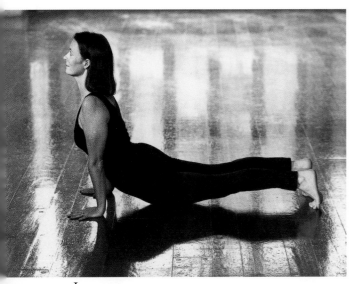

I

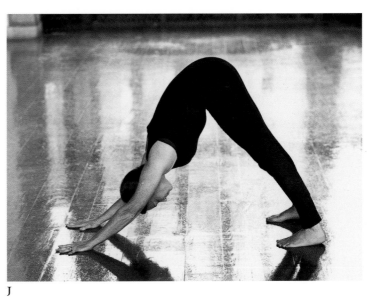

J

N

O

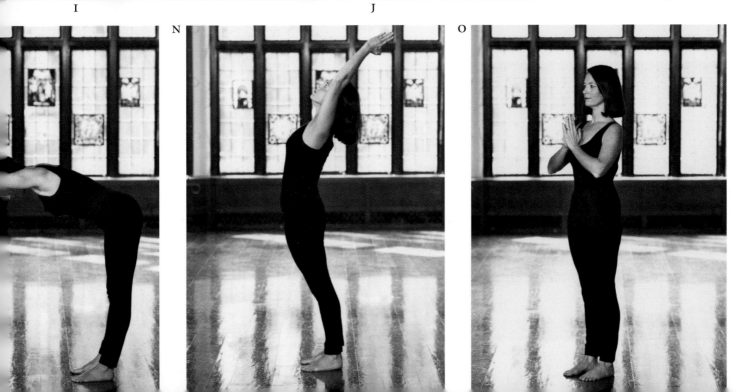

KNEE-DOWN TWIST

Body Benefits:

➤ Rotates and flexes spinal column

➤ Stretches waist, hips, shoulders, and neck

➤ Removes stiffness from shoulders and neck

➤ Strengthens spinal nerves

➤ Increases flexibility in hip joints

➤ Stimulates digestion and elimination

➤ Increases blood supply to spine

➤ Releases tension from body and mind

When to avoid this posture If you have disc problems or abdominal hernia, do not practice the Knee-Down Twist.

Yoga Tip Flexibility comes with practice. Come into each stretch or twist more deeply on the exhalation. When you exhale, you open up and let go. Notice when your mind "stiffens." Does your body tighten up too? By developing the Spiritual Muscle of Flexibility, you will also strengthen your ability in a wide range of other areas of your life, from yard work to stair climbing, from your sex life to your sporting life.

Let's begin:

1. Begin by lying on your back with your legs stretched out on the ground.

2. Bring your right knee up toward the chest. Place your hands a few inches below your right knee and hug the knee into the chest. The legs are totally relaxed; let your arms do the work.

3. Release your hands, stretching your arms out to the sides in a T. Keep the right knee bent and place the right foot—heel, arch, or toes, whatever is comfortable—on top of the left knee.

4. On an exhalation, lift the right hip and drop the right knee toward your left side. Allow the right knee to come as close to the floor as possible without lifting the right shoulder.

5. To complete the stretch, turn your head to face the right hand. You may choose to place the left hand on the right bent knee to come into a deeper stretch.

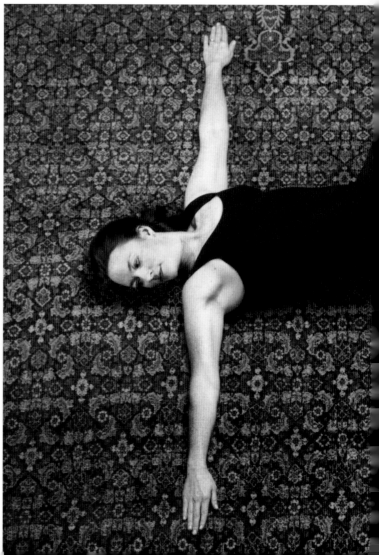

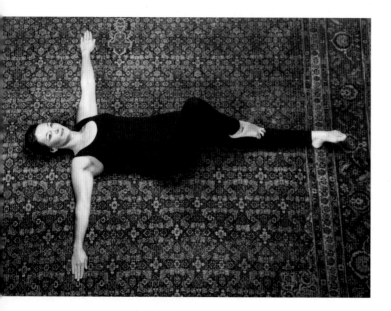

6. Take five to ten full and deep breaths in this posture.

7. Bring the right knee back up to face the ceiling, and then stretch it out along the floor to meet your left leg.

8. Repeat steps 2–7 bending the *left* knee.

9. After twisting to both sides, hug both knees to your chest with your hands clasping just below the knees.

10. Slowly rock along your lower back from left to right, as though you are wearing a belt and rocking along the place that the belt would touch the ground.

11. Release the hug and lower both legs back down.

12. Take a moment with eyes closed to check in and notice any changes, shifts, or parts of the body that feel more agile.

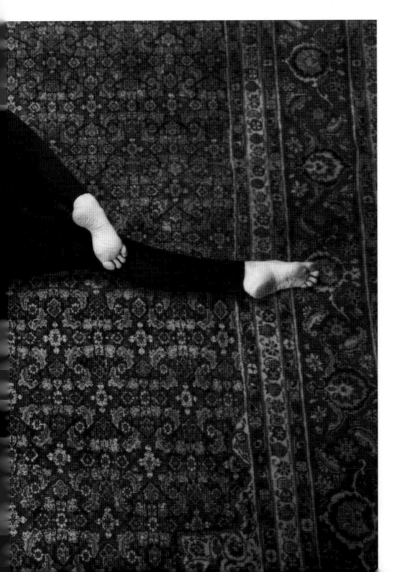

CREATE YOUR OWN POSTURE FOR FLEXIBILITY

Let's begin:

1. Practice the formal postures before creating your own.

2. Begin in Proper Standing Alignment with your eyes closed. Take several deep breaths.

3. Imagine that your body is incredibly flexible. In your mind's eye, see yourself bending and stretching with the agility of a gymnast or a dancer.

4. Sense every cell in your body moving. Feel your entire being as limber, elastic, and vital.

5. Keep your eyes closed as you allow your body to move very slowly in whatever direction or manner it chooses. Reach your arms, stretch your legs, bend at the waist or knees—whatever feels best.

6. Let your body move in slow motion for several minutes. When you find a position that you want to hold, stop moving. Stay in this position for several breaths. Open your eyes if you wish.

7. Make a note of the posture you have created. Draw or write about it in your yoga journal. Create an affirmation about your Flexibility goals that you can state when you are in your posture. Add this posture to your regular practice. Or change it if you want to—that's what Flexibility is all about!

THREE-PART BREATH

Body Benefits:

➤ Brings flexibility to rib cage

➤ Lowers blood pressure

➤ Relieves and reduces respiratory problems and helps develop immunity to them

➤ Increases lung capacity and efficiency

➤ Calms and energizes both body and mind

➤ Restores oxygen if you are out of breath from anger, fear, or any vigorous activity

➤ Strengthens diaphragm

➤ Relaxes abdominal, middle, and upper torso tension

➤ Improves digestion and elimination

Breathing Tip The stress of everyday life can form a straightjacket on our breathing apparatus. Unless we are careful, the breath can become constricted, shallow, and concentrated in our upper chest only. When we breathe only in the upper part of the chest, it's as though we own a three-bedroom house but live in only one room. The Three-Part Breath gives us access to the other rooms so that we have more choices, more room for growth, and greater flexibility.

When to avoid this technique The Three-Part Breath is safe for everyone. If at any time you feel that you are out of breath, hyperventilating, or straining, simply stop. *Do* avoid such full breathing near polluted areas, chemicals, vehicle exhaust on busy streets, and at any other time you question the air quality.

Let's begin:

1. Come into Proper Sitting Alignment.

2. Relax deeply by taking several full breaths.

3. When you pour a glass of water, the water fills up the bottom of the glass first, right? For this exercise, imagine that your entire torso is a giant glass. Instead of water, you will be filling and emptying this glass with air.

4. Take an inhalation and begin to fill your imaginary glass with air. Place one hand on your lower belly to feel it expand as the "bottom" fills up.

5. Continue inhaling, feeling the rib cage expand as the glass is filled to the middle. You may wish to place your other hand on your outer rib cage to note its expansion.

6. Finally, fill the glass to the top by letting the air flow into your upper chest. Bring your hand from the rib cage up to the sternum (breast bone).

7. Now that your glass is full, begin to slowly exhale. Let the air "pour" out of your body, releasing it from your upper chest first.

8. Continue exhaling as you empty your middle chest. You may move your upper hand back to the rib cage to feel how it relaxes inward as the air exits.

9. Finally, empty the glass. Pull the lower belly in toward your spine. This will push the remaining air out.

10. Steps 4–9 equal one round. Repeat in fluid, rhythmic movements for five to ten more rounds.

11. You are filled with both breath and spirit. When you are done, sit quietly feeling the expansive Flexibility in your breath.

ANCHORS AWEIGH!

Let's begin:

1. Come into the Corpse Pose. Breathe deeply.

2. Call to mind an unresolved experience in your life. It might be a situation in which you feel stuck or have little choice. It could be a personal habit, a belief, or a relationship issue.

3. As if you were in a dream, imagine that you are on a magic boat in the ocean. You are completely safe here throughout your journey. The anchor is down so the boat stays in one place. Sitting in your boat, begin to focus on your unresolved situation. Check in with your thoughts and feelings about it.

4. The rope for the anchor is at your feet. Pick up the rope and begin pulling up the anchor. As it emerges from the water, you are surprised to find a beautiful treasure box on the end of it. Inside a note reads: "Wherever you go, ask this question: 'What can I do about my situation?'"

5. As you gaze over the side of your magic boat, you see your favorite sea animals swimming alongside. They invite you in for a swim. While you play in the water, you remember the note. You ask, "What can I do about my situation?" The answer may come through words, a feeling, or a gift.

6. Take a moment to receive their response. It may come right now or at a later time.

7. Thank the creatures for their help and climb back aboard your boat. Put the answer the sea animals gave you into your treasure box. If it was a spoken message, whisper it into the treasure box and close the lid.

8. Your boat now brings you right up to the shore of a tiny island. Get out and walk along the beautiful beach. Ask the beach, "What can I do about my situation?"

9. As you walk, you notice up ahead that an answer has been written in the sand. What does it say? Now return to your boat. As it pulls away and heads back out to sea, whisper into your treasure box the message you saw in the sand.

10. Suddenly, you hear voices calling your name. When you look back toward the shore, you see smiling natives paddling a canoe toward you. When they reach your boat, ask them "What can I do about my situation?"

11. The canoers give you a gift. Thank them for the present and place it in your treasure box.

12. The wind carries you farther still. The boat brings you to a place where the waves are bigger than before. A very wise and special Being is riding the waves. The Being signals for you to join in. You spend several moments riding the waves and enjoying yourself.

13. Ask this special Being your question: "What can I do about my situation?" Listen carefully for the message to come in any shape or form. Place the message in your treasure box.

14. Your boat retraces its route. You pass the natives, the tiny island, the playful sea animals, past the spot you were first anchored, and back to harbor.

15. Bring your treasure box ashore. Take a moment to consider these four gifts of guidance. Imagine yourself in the original situation. What new perspectives have you gained?

16. Keep your treasures with you as you begin to return from your adventures. Feel your body on the floor. Deepen your breath.

17. At your own pace, gently roll over onto one side. Hug your knees close to your chest, and bring yourself into a seated position. Allow your eyes to open.

18. Take ten minutes to write or draw any new insights you may have gained. Who were your guides? What did your treasure box look like? How do you feel? Are you better able to handle your situation? Do you feel more flexible in your way of looking at it? Respect your experience and all it has to offer.

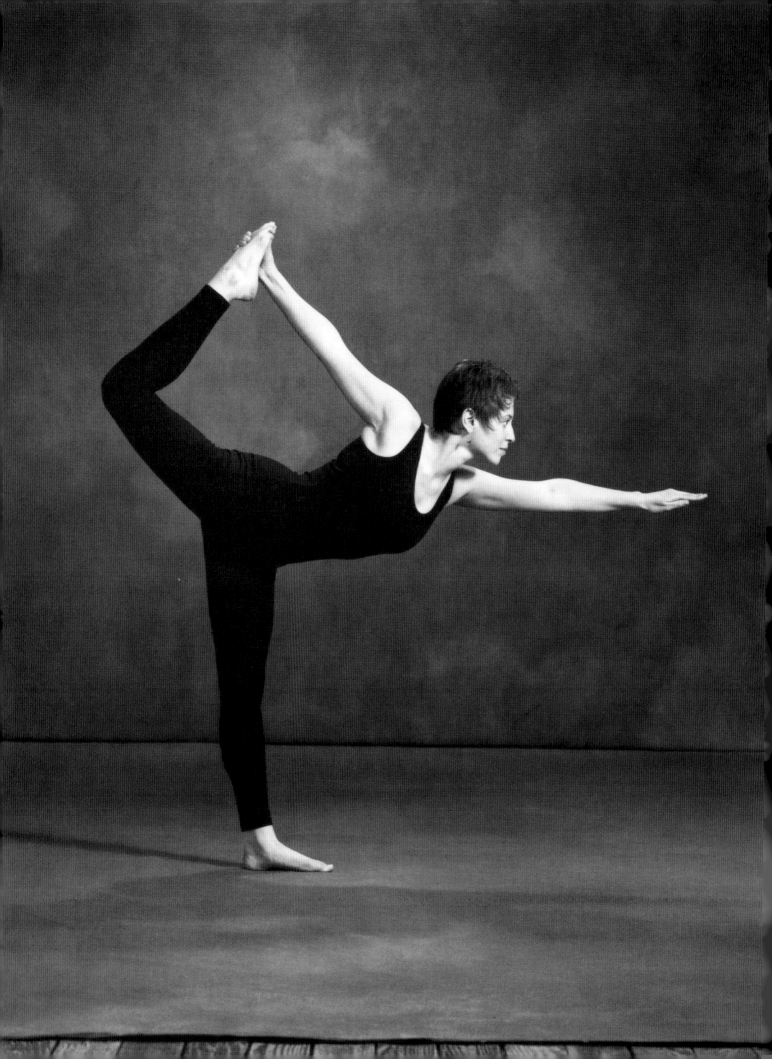

BALANCE

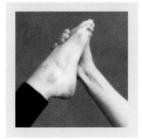

Life is a balancing act. We need sun, but too much can give us sunstroke or skin cancer. We need exercise, but not to the point of exhaustion. Work is important, but play must be a part of our lives as well. We must bring all parts of ourselves into Balance in order to feel centered. Our bodies need as much attention as our minds, which must be nurtured with as much care as our spirits. (And while we're at it, wouldn't it be nice to have a balanced checkbook?)

We do not always feel balanced in our daily lives. Sometimes, certain parts of our lives weigh more and we need to adjust. We might need to swing back and forth on the pendulum in order to eventually find center. It is within a calm and relaxed state of body and mind that we flow most easily with life's changes and challenges. When we find our Balance on a higher level, we liberate the spirit.

Ancient Chinese and Greek traditions promote Balance as the key to good health and a long life. The Chinese embrace the law of *yin* and *yang*—two opposing forces that make up everything in the universe. Health is restored by bringing excessive or deficient yin and yang into harmony. This balances the vital energy in the body, known as *qi*.

The Taoist religion sprang from the Chinese people's observations of opposites working together in harmony. Rather than seeing the opposites of the universe in conflict, the Chinese viewed the move-

ment from night to day and winter to summer and other natural cycles as forming a rhythmic union. The *Tao*, which means way or process, is a path of Balance both for humans and for the universe.

In Taoism, everything must be in Balance. Things that are out of Balance are cured with sacred charms. Even today, large business developers and private home owners call upon the expertise of special designers to Balance with nature the elements of working or living environments. These *feng shui* designers Balance out extremes and excesses so that inhabitants will find harmony within themselves and every aspect of their lives.

The great Greek physician Hippocrates believed that the four fluids that compose the body (blood, phlegm, yellow bile, and black bile) must be in Balance for health to exist. Hippocrates looked to nature to find the wisdom of healing.

The Greeks personified the Balance of the seasons in the myth of Demeter, the great earth

It is impossible to practice yoga effectively if you eat or sleep either too much or too little. But if you are moderate in eating, playing, sleeping, and staying awake, and avoid extremes in everything you do, you will see that these yoga practices eliminate all of your pain and suffering.

—BHAGAVAD GITA, CHAPTER 6, VERSES 16 AND 17

mother and goddess of the harvest. One day, Hades, the god of the Underworld, stole Demeter's daughter, Persephone. Demeter was so grief stricken that she abandoned the earth, allowing the vegetation to dry up. Before Persephone was freed to return to her mother, Hades tricked her into eating pomegranate seeds. Now she must spend part of each year in the Underworld. And so Persephone lives with Hades throughout the cold, icy months while the earth is frozen. She returns to live with her mother when Spring arrives and the world is renewed.

In all cultures, nature teaches us the rhythm of Balance. Even a small garden contains the cycles of life: a time to plant, to grow, to harvest, to decay, and to regenerate.

Just as the earth finds its Balance through seasonal cycles, we can find our Balance through yoga. Even the word *hatha*, Sanskrit for the physical path of yoga, demonstrates Balance: *ha* means "sun" and *tha* means "moon." Yoga embodies the principles of symmetry. Whatever you practice on the right side, repeat on the left. Forward bends compliment backbends. Twisting to one side invites twisting on the other. None of the poses are static; you are constantly readjusting. Visual focus is the key to maintaining equilibrium. To the extent that you concentrate on a fixed point, your body will also remain steady.

While your visual focus should be one pointed, your weight should feel as though it were distributed among many points. If you are standing on one foot, for example, instead of feeling the foot as one point, imagine three places on the foot—the big toe, the little toe, and the heel forming a balanced triangle. This way, your foot will feel like a tripod instead of a one-legged table. Developing the Spiritual Muscle of Balance helps us experience life in a fluid, congruous, and graceful way.

Postures for Balance Try the Tree, Standing Knee Balance, King/Queen of the Dancers, Table Balance, and Standing Stick to help you find a state of equipoise. Play with Balance without getting overly serious about it.

Breathing Lesson for Balance The Balancing Breath is a beautiful technique that you can practice daily to bring a sense of stability into your life. It helps bring both sides of the brain into harmony.

Visualization for Balance What would it feel like to have a perfectly balanced day? Try this exercise and see how it plays out in your day-to-day experience.

To be in Balance, it's essential to have the breath in Balance. When we're angry, the exhalation tends to be stronger than the inhalation. When we're sad, the inhalation tends to be stronger than the exhalation. When we're feeling fear, we don't breathe much at all. By bringing the breath back into Balance . . . it helps bring our life back into Balance.

—DAN MILLMAN, AUTHOR OF *WAY OF THE PEACEFUL WARRIOR*

FROM "NEW DIMENSIONS" PUBLIC RADIO INTERVIEW

YOGA STORY FOR BALANCE: STEPHEN COPE

Sweating, a rapid heart rate, and butterflies in the stomach are just a few of the very real reactions many of us experience during a public performance. When fear gets the better of us, we get thrown off Balance. Stephen Cope got himself back on center using the Balancing Breath.

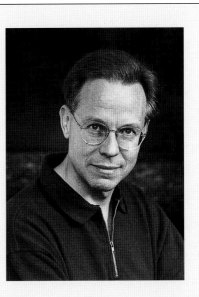

Last year my piano teacher talked me into playing a concert with her. I still don't know quite how she did this. I don't like playing in public; I get anxious. I must not have been paying attention when I agreed, at the beginning of the year, to play a couple of piano pieces for four hands with her at an evening celebrating the work of Franz Schubert.

As the date for the performance drew closer, I was beyond nervous. I've studied the piano since I was seven, but I've always been just an amateur. This was to be a professional concert. In the weeks leading up to the event, I pulled out all of my yoga resources to see if any of them could make a dent in my anxiety. Guess what? They worked! My years of practicing yoga were about to pay off in my real life.

In order to perform effectively, a pianist needs to have a balanced combination of excitement and calm. Some nervousness is good. It brings an edge to the music. Too much nervousness, though, is the kiss of death. It constricts the muscles of the hands and tightens the feelings as well.

I was extremely nervous until I discovered the one practice that helped create the Balance I needed: the Balancing Breath. Its effects were practically miraculous. After seven to ten minutes of simple alternate-nostril breathing, I had plenty of energy, clarity of mind, *and* equanimity.

As I awaited my turn to perform, I tried to do the Balancing Breath unobtrusively. This is not easy, since it requires placing your hands on your nose for long periods of time and looks decidedly weird and antisocial. But I needed the calming and invigorating effects of this practice more than I needed the approval of the audience sitting behind (and presumably watching) me. So, there I was: "Breathe in, breathe out, thumb, fourth finger . . ."

How did the performance go? Well, my piano teacher is still speaking to me—and still teaching me! I'm sure it wouldn't have gone nearly as well without my secret weapon.

To attain spirituality is to realize that the whole universe is one symphony in which every individual is one note. His happiness lies in becoming perfectly harmonious with the symphony of the universe. It is not by following a certain religion that makes one spiritual, or having a certain belief, or being a fanatic in regard to one idea, or by becoming too good to live in this world. . . .
Ultimate good is harmony itself.

—HAZRAT INAYAT KHAN,
FROM *THE MYSTICISM OF SOUND AND MUSIC*

TREE

Body Benefits:

➤ Improves posture and balance

➤ Focuses and clears mind

➤ Improves concentration

➤ Flexes ankle, knee, and hip joints

➤ Tones and strengthens legs

➤ Strengthens internal abdominal muscles

➤ Improves breathing

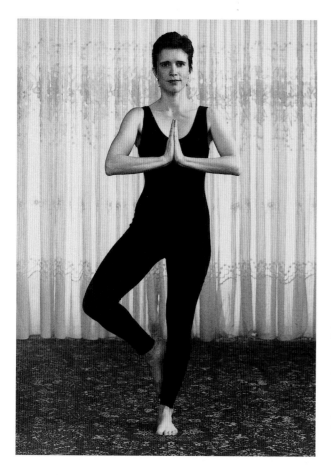

I have become attached to practicing yoga. It feels so good to let my mind and body be equal with one another. It has changed my entire being.

— IRENE LOIZOU, YOGA STUDENT

Let's begin:

1. Begin in Proper Standing Alignment, maintaining your visual focus on a tree or a point on the wall in front of you.

2. Shift all of your weight onto your left foot, so that your belly button and nose are in line with and directly over the left foot.

3. Play with your Balance for a moment: lift the right foot off the ground and use it to explore the space around you at a low level.

4. When you've found your Balance, lift the right foot and place it on the inside of the left ankle (for beginners), the inside of the left knee, or the inside of the upper left leg (more advanced). The right knee should not be in front of the body. Instead, keep it bent and turned to the right.

5. Bring your palms together in prayer position.

6. BREATHE!!! Sometimes when you are in deep concentration, you hold your breath. Try to keep the breath moving smoothly.

7. Be aware of your body alignment. It helps to stay conscious of good alignment while you are in the posture.

8. If you feel steady, you can raise your arms overhead in steeple position. Your palms remain together, fingers interlaced, and the pointer fingers aim directly at the ceiling.

9. Hold, breathe, focus, and relax.

10. To release, lower your hands back into prayer position in front of your heart.

11. Lower your arms to the sides. Lower the right foot back to the floor.

12. Allow your eyes to close for a moment and check in. What did it feel like to Balance? Do you feel balanced in your daily life? What does it feel like now to Balance on both feet? Notice the difference between the two sides of your body.

13. Repeat the Tree standing on your right foot.

14. After you have practiced the Tree on both sides, close your eyes again to notice how you feel and what is happening in the mind.

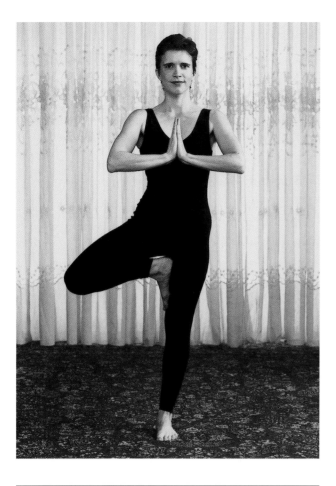

I used to run from one thing to another, seemingly putting out fires. I can now stop. Through a few quiet minutes of yoga, I can get centered and restore my Balance.

—CAROL ZAINO, YOGA STUDENT

STANDING KNEE BALANCE

Body Benefits:

➤ Strengthens back and leg muscles, hip joints

➤ Tones abdominal organs

➤ Stimulates digestion, circulation, and respiration

➤ Strengthens back

➤ Builds heat and energy throughout body

➤ Prepares body for King/Queen of the Dancers

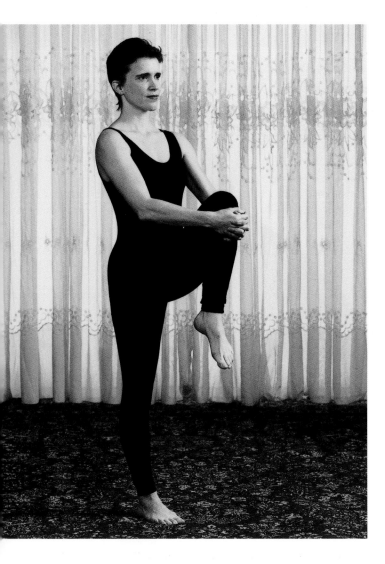

Let's begin:

1. Begin in Proper Standing Alignment. Keep your focus on one point on the wall ahead of you.

2. Lift your right foot up and gain a sense of Balance standing on your left leg.

3. Keep your spine straight. Reach down and clasp the underside of your right thigh and hug up to your chest.

4. Now reach around to the outside of the bent knee and clasp a firm hold. As you draw your knee in close to your body, be sure to maintain good alignment. Don't lean over the bent leg.

5. Hold for five to ten breaths.

6. Gently release the bent leg.

7. Close your eyes and notice the difference between the right and left sides of the body.

8. Repeat steps 1–6 on the opposite side.

9. After you have completed both sides, stand in stillness with your eyes closed and experience the satisfying feeling of Balance.

Yoga Tip Practice on a flat surface—either a hardwood floor or a thin rug. Balanced alignment differs in some respects from traditional Proper Standing Alignment. Before you lift your knee into the fullest expression of the posture, bring your standing-leg toes, navel, and nose into alignment. Imagine a continuous support running through these three points. Spread your toes, as they are there for Balance. Always activate the abdominals in balancing poses by lifting these muscles. They are the key to supporting your lower back as well.

On the Job: Balance Your Work Day and Build Productivity

Yoga during the work day is not as crazy as it sounds. Many studies have shown a relationship between taking short, relaxing breaks and working in a more productive, efficient, and energized way. True, you probably cannot take a full hour out of your morning, change your clothes, and find a quiet, comfortable area conducive to a complete yoga practice. However, there are many easy and simple ways to add minipractice sessions into your schedule. Balance is the key to effective yoga breaks:

1. If your primary work involves sitting, stand up and practice a posture or two. If you've been in one position for a long time, move around and shake the stiffness out.

2. After more than an hour of heavy visual work, whether at a computer or not, close your eyes and practice Neck Openers, Face Massage, or rest your head on your desk. If you spend a lot of your day talking, take a break by listening to soothing music.

3. Explore other uses for your desk chair. Use it as a prop for a standing balancing pose. Stand behind the chair, rest your hands on top of it, and come forward into the Jackknife. Dave Garland, President of MP Systems Inc., a computer consultant, is the "King of Chair Yoga." When others are running for the three o'clock coffee break, Dave energizes his body and mind in the privacy of his office. He practices modified Spinal Twists and Rag Dolls. He has also been known to practice the Shoulder Opener in meetings. "It's unobtrusive, and it's better than falling asleep at the conference table."

4. Vary your scenery. If you don't have windows in your office, take a short stretch break outside. Practice the Tree and notice the seasonal colors.

5. Get some air—and not just by going outside. Often when we're focused on details or overwhelmed with too much to do, we hold the breath. Set your watch to go off at every hour, and take a thirty-second breathing break to increase oxygen in your system.

6. Balance solitary moments by inviting coworkers to join you. You may wish to teach them a simple pose. They may be skeptical at first, but soon they'll be asking you for guidance.

7. If you've been surrounded by serious problems, take a lighthearted break. Try the Lion or practice a miniversion of Polarity Relaxation. With each exhalation, imagine the heaviness flowing out of your body.

8. In Ann McGee-Cooper's *You Don't Have to Go Home from Work Exhausted*, she says, "Be sure to balance your work with refreshing, invigorating play." For example, if you have a long meeting to sit through, free your feet from the jail of your shoes, and wiggle them around underneath the conference table. Or take a thirty-second break outdoors before the meeting starts and practice the Breath of Fire so that you can remain alert and enthusiastic.

9. Once you complete a project of any size, reward yourself with a yoga break. Spend two minutes standing in Warrior I or Warrior II to savor your triumphant accomplishment *before* moving on to the next goal.

10. The right side of the brain controls the left side of the body, and the left side of the brain controls the right side of the body. Before starting a new task, determine what sorts of skills you will need. Studies show that breathing through the *left* nostril (and blocking the right) stimulates the right brain, which is responsible for creativity, as in design work. If you need to focus on more linear activities such as speaking or writing (controlled by the left brain), breathe in and out through the *right* nostril. Or for full integration practice the Balancing Breath.

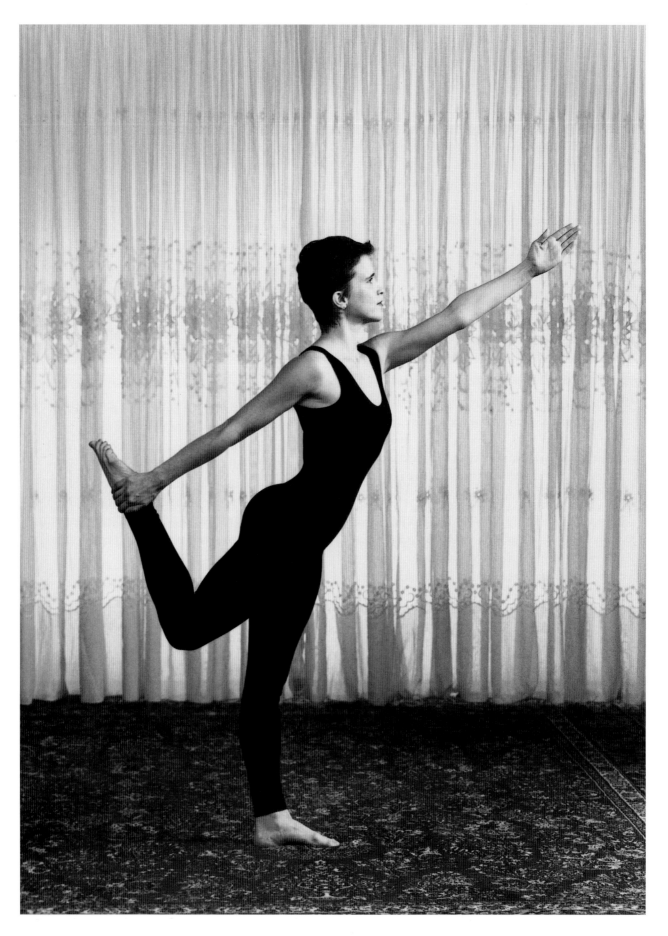

King/Queen of the Dancers

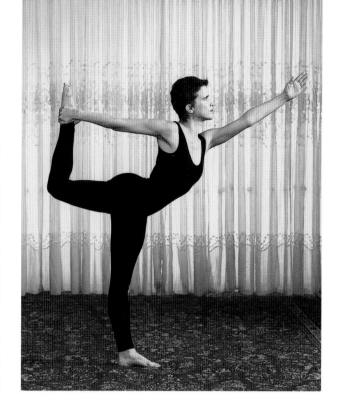

Body Benefits:

➤ Brings fresh blood to internal organs and glands

➤ Tones abdomen, thighs, arms, hips, buttocks, and legs

➤ Expands lung capacity and strengthens chest

➤ Promotes proper kidney functioning

➤ Energizes endocrine system including adrenals, pancreas, thyroid, and gonads

➤ Improves digestion and relieves constipation

➤ Invigorates and warms body

➤ Increases shoulder and spinal flexibility and strength

Let's begin:

1. Start in Proper Standing Alignment. Your eyes are fixed on one point on the wall ahead of you, about eye level.

2. Shift all your weight onto the left leg. Engage the standing left leg by lifting the thigh. Bend the right knee and lift the right foot behind you and up toward your buttocks. Reach back with your right hand and grab the outside or inside of the right foot.

3. Raise the left arm out in front of you. Align the body by bringing your knees close together and your hips squared forward.

4. Beginners can remain here to practice Balance. When you are ready, move on to step 5.

5. Rather then using the arm to pull the leg up, *slowly press* the right foot into the right hand as you shift the torso forward. Go only as far as your body feels ready to. Be sure to keep your bent leg moving *up* rather than out to the side. (Eventually your torso will be parallel with the ground. If you are facing a mirror, your elevated foot will appear right above your head.)

6. As you shift forward, your gaze will follow a steady path downward so that it remains at eye level.

7. Hold for three to ten breaths depending upon your level of comfort and ability.

8. To release, *slowly* lift the torso back to an upright position. Simultaneously release the right leg to the floor as you lower the arms to your sides.

9. Take a deep breath and exhale with your eyes closed before switching sides. Repeat steps 1–9, balancing on the right leg.

10. When you have completed both sides, stand in stillness for a moment with the eyes closed and feel the effects of this powerful posture.

Yoga Tip You will probably find that you can Balance more easily on one side than the other. If you are right handed, you may find it easier to maintain your equilibrium on your left side to Balance out your dominance. You will surely notice that your Balance is better on some days than on others. If you fall out of Balance, who cares? This elegant pose may remind you of a statue in an ancient garden. If you find yourself hopping around as if on a pogo stick, think of yourself as a moving statue. Try not to take yourself too seriously—don't use yoga as an opportunity to judge yourself!

TABLE BALANCE

Body Benefits:

➤ Strengthens, elongates and aligns spinal column

➤ Strengthens wrists, arms, shoulders, abdominals, and legs

➤ Tones hips, thighs, and buttocks

➤ Strengthens legs, spine, shoulders, arms, and hips

➤ Improves circulation

➤ Expands lung capacity

➤ Helps develop coordination

Yoga Tip Balancing is fun! Have you ever watched a juggler? Her job is to Balance the balls in a way that is entertaining. Two favorite circus shows are the tightrope walkers and stilt walkers who must steady and center themselves to find equilibrium. When a seal balances a ball on the end of her nose, the audience roars with applause. Delight in playing with Balance in your yoga practice.

Before yoga, I was busy doing everything at once—my mind was in three places, my body switching back and forth, my soul going along for the ride. After yoga, I feel like all three are balanced and unified as one.

—GLENN SIEGEL, YOGA STUDENT

Let's begin:

1. Start in the Table position on all fours. Your hands are directly under your shoulders and your knees are directly under your hips. Your gaze is downward so that your head is in line with your spine.

2. Lift the left leg straight out behind you so that it is at the same height as your spine. For beginners, this may be as far as you take the Table Balance.

3. If you feel ready to move on, lift the right arm straight out in front of you, at the same height as your spine. You can keep your gaze downward or look out over the outstretched hand.

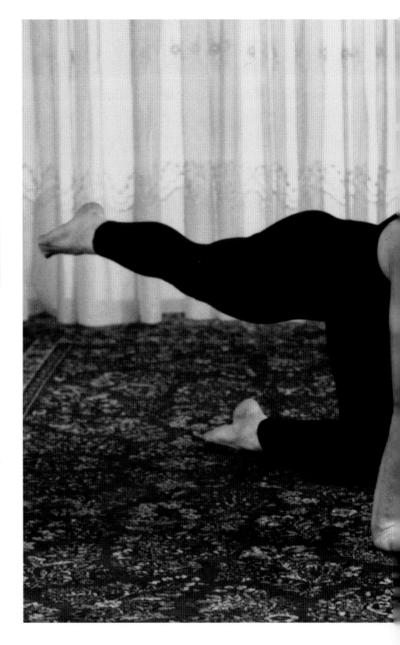

4. Be sure to breathe deeply as you reach the opposite arm and leg away from the center of your body. You may need to make micromovements to find your equilibrium.

5. To release, simultaneously bring the arm and leg back into the Table position.

6. Repeat steps 1–5 with the right leg and left arm.

7. Once you have completed both sides, remain in the Table position for several moments. Absorb the sensations present in your body.

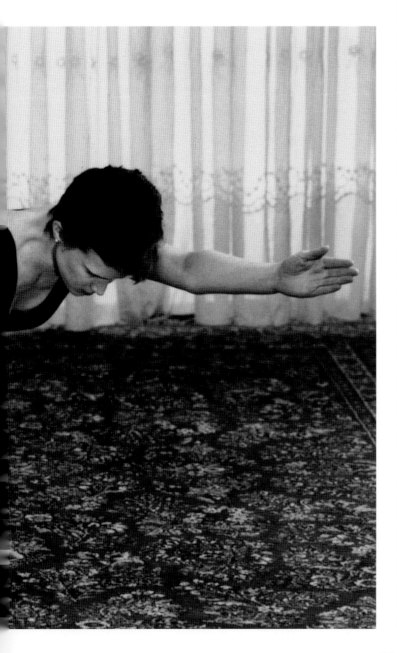

CREATE YOUR OWN POSTURE FOR BALANCE

1. Practice the formal postures before you create your own.

2. Begin in a standing position with your eyes closed. Take several long, deep breaths.

3. Call to mind a symbol that you can adopt as your icon for Balance. The astrological sign Libra epitomizes Balance. Scales are the symbol of this sun sign and represent harmony and symmetry. Choose whatever symbol works best for you. Hold it in the forefront of your mind.

4. Acknowledge your body and all of the systems within it that form the vital Balance of keeping you alive and healthy.

5. Notice what it feels like to be steady on two feet. Develop a breathing pattern that feels balanced to you. Sense a strong center within you—as if that is the only thing that matters, and all other appendages are just auxiliary parts that can move about freely without interrupting your center.

6. Open your eyes softly and begin to play with different ways of balancing: come up onto your toes, lift one leg in the air, kneel down and Balance on your forearms and knees, or any other way that you can imagine. Again, let your movements come from a strong center.

7. Once you find a position that you want to hold, stay there and breathe. If you want, close your eyes. (Not being able to focus can make balancing more difficult, however.)

8. Make a note of the posture you have created and give it a name. Add it to your regular practice, and create an affirmation that Balance exists in your life. Reinforce the meaning of this posture by practicing it when you feel balanced. Once it becomes natural for you, practice it also when you lack harmony.

Body Benefits:

➤ Tones hips, thighs, abdominals, and buttocks

➤ Improves posture

➤ Energizes entire system

➤ Strengthens legs, spine, shoulders, arms, and hips

➤ Improves circulation and strengthens heart

➤ Expands lung capacity

STANDING STICK

Let's begin:

1. Come into Proper Standing Alignment. Keep your eyes fixed on one point on the wall ahead of you, about eye level.

2. Raise your arms overhead with the palms and fingers together. Keep the shoulders relaxed and down.

3. Step forward with your right foot and lift the left leg up slightly so that your foot is poised with

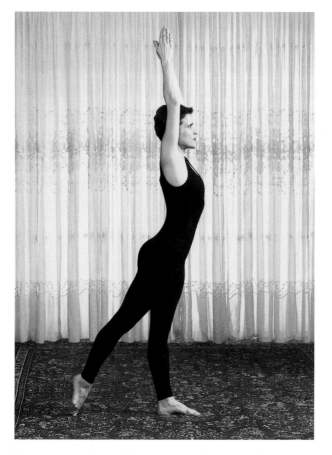

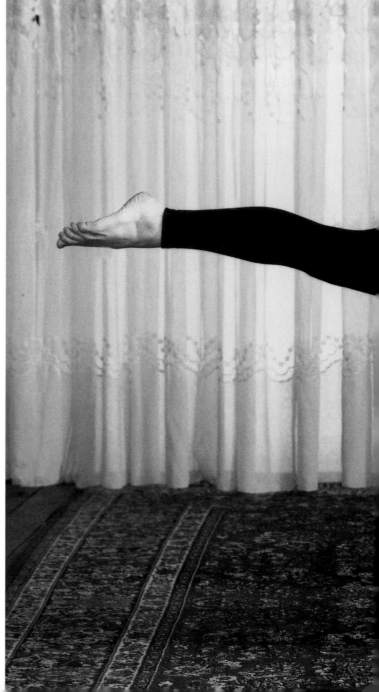

Yoga Tip Try using props to help you gain a sense of Balance. A wall, a chair, or a door can be a supportive friend when learning the art of steadiness. I trained myself to do many of the balancing poses while holding onto the towel rack of my oven door. (I recommend keeping the oven *off*.)

toes touching the floor. Beginners can remain here to practice Balance.

4. When you are ready to move into a fuller expression of the posture, raise your left leg out behind you as you simultaneously shift the torso forward with a *flat* back. Move slowly and keep the hip bones facing forward and then down, rather than opening out to the left side. Your gaze will shift down as you come forward.

5. Focus on lengthening the body with the toes reaching away from the fingertips. Imagine that your body is one long line resting on the "stick" of your right leg.

6. Eventually your torso and left leg will be parallel to the ground.

7. To release, slowly lower the left leg as you return to center, keeping the arms overhead. Take a deep breath in and out. As you feel ready, shift to the other side.

8. Repeat steps 1–7 balancing on the left leg.

9. When you have completed both sides, assume Proper Standing Alignment with your eyes closed. Notice how you feel.

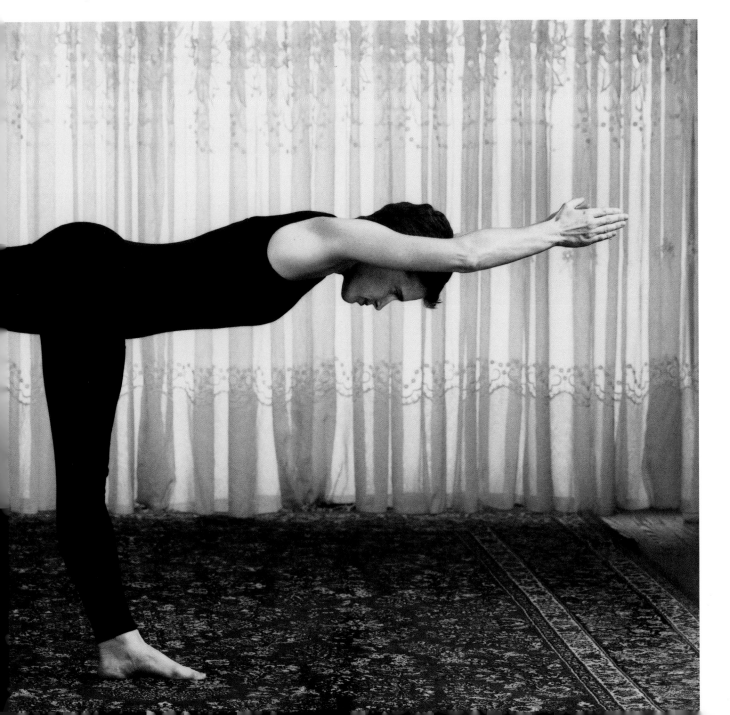

BALANCING BREATH

Body Benefits:

➤ Restores natural breathing rhythm

➤ Improves blood oxygenation

➤ Calms nerves and stills mind

➤ Balances hemispheres of brain

➤ Helps those who suffer from fatigue and insomnia

➤ Aids sinus problems

Let's begin:

1. Come into Proper Sitting Alignment. Remember not to strain or force the breath.

2. Bring your hands into what is known as the Vishnu Mudra: the right palm faces your body with your second and third fingers tucked into your palm.

3. Bring the thumb up to close off the right nostril.

4. Exhale completely through the left nostril.

5. Inhale slowly through the left nostril.

6. Close off the left nostril with the fourth and fifth fingers. Release the thumb from the right nostril as you exhale slowly.

7. Inhale gently through the right nostril.

8. Close off the air from the right nostril using the thumb, and release the fourth and fifth fingers from the left nostril, exhaling gently.

9. This sequence is one round. Remember: there is a slight pause between the inhalations and the exhalations. Repeat for ten to fifteen rounds.

10. When you are finished, lower the right hand into your lap and notice the balancing effects of this breath.

When to avoid this breathing lesson If you have a history of nervous disorders, high blood pressure, heart disease, or strokes, or if you are pregnant, consult your health care practitioner before using this technique.

Yoga Tip This technique is said to Balance the two hemispheres of the brain. A healthy person alternates breathing dominance between the right and left nostrils about every two hours. However, this natural flow often becomes unbalanced. Place your hand or a small mirror underneath your nostrils and see which one is dominant right now. Though we use both sides of the brain, we are naturally dominant in one side (just as we are more right-handed than left-handed or vice-versa). The left side of the brain is responsible for our rational, logical, and linear thinking. Creative, divergent thinking is the job of the right brain. When these hemispheres are a cooperative team, the rewards are unlimited.

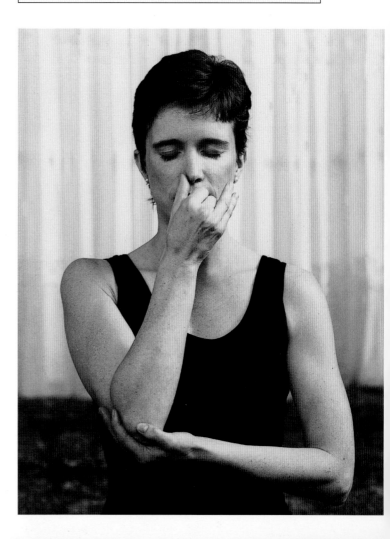

BALANCED DAY

Let's begin:

1. Come into the Corpse Pose. Breathe deeply.

2. In your imagination, call to mind a typical day out of your present life. Begin with how you wake up. Do you use an alarm, a family member, or your natural body clock?

3. What is your first meal of the day? Mentally review all of the ingredients. Be specific. How much time do you allow yourself to eat? Do you feel nurtured by this food? Is it a nutritionally balanced meal?

4. Do you bathe yourself in the morning? Do you lovingly caress your body as a form of self-massage or just get the job done—splash some soap on yourself and jump out?

5. What is the quality of your commute to work? Do you listen to the radio? If so, what: local news reports, relaxing music, an inspirational speaker? Does the commute bring anything special to your day?

6. Review the typical morning experience. What emotions come up during the pre-lunch hours? With whom do you communicate and how? Do you enjoy these people?

7. What sort of break, if any, do you allow yourself? If you do take a breather, do you go outdoors? Drink coffee?

8. Lunch time arrives. Do you eat? If so, be specific about the contents. Are you alone or with others? Is the conversation recreational or professional? Does lunch time feel like a break or does it continue the mental process? Do you feel that you digest this food well? Do you digest your experiences well?

9. What happens in the afternoon? Are you typically energized or fatigued? Do you stay behind a chair at a desk, or do you move around? Are you in contact with your family? Your feelings? How could you bring Balance into your afternoon experience?

10. What is the commute home like? Again, are you alone or with others? How do you feel at this time of day? What would make this part of your day feel more balanced?

11. What is the first thing that you do when you arrive home? Whom do you see? Do you take time for yourself to unwind, or jump right into the next activity? Is that activity pleasurable for you?

12. What is the dinner experience like? Do you and your family have any special rituals? Do you light candles or spend a few moments in silence before you eat? Do you eat a balanced meal?

13. What happens between dinner and bedtime? Do you watch television? If so, which programs? Whom do you spend time with and how?

14. Do you have any bedtime rituals? Do you read? Pray? Take a bath? Listen to relaxing music? Watch the world news? Take a brief walk? Spend time with your kids? How do you usually feel at this point in the day? Ready for bed? Exhausted? Satisfied?

15. In reviewing a typical day, what stands out for you? Are there any significant gaps? Do you feel balanced, or is there part of you that is not receiving attention? Do you allow time for both doing and being? Do you Balance indoor time with enjoying nature? Time thinking and time feeling? Play and work? Reflection and action? Social time and time for yourself?

16. Now go back and review your typical day and fill in simple remedies for creating Balance in your day. Start at the time that you wake up and finish at bedtime. Play out these new ideas as if you were watching them take place on a movie screen inside your mind. See yourself successfully mastering the art of Balance. Make sure your new ideas are do-able and accessible.

17. Slowly roll over onto one side. Gently draw your body back up into a comfortable seated position. Notice your attitude and take your emotional temperature. Allow your eyes to open slowly.

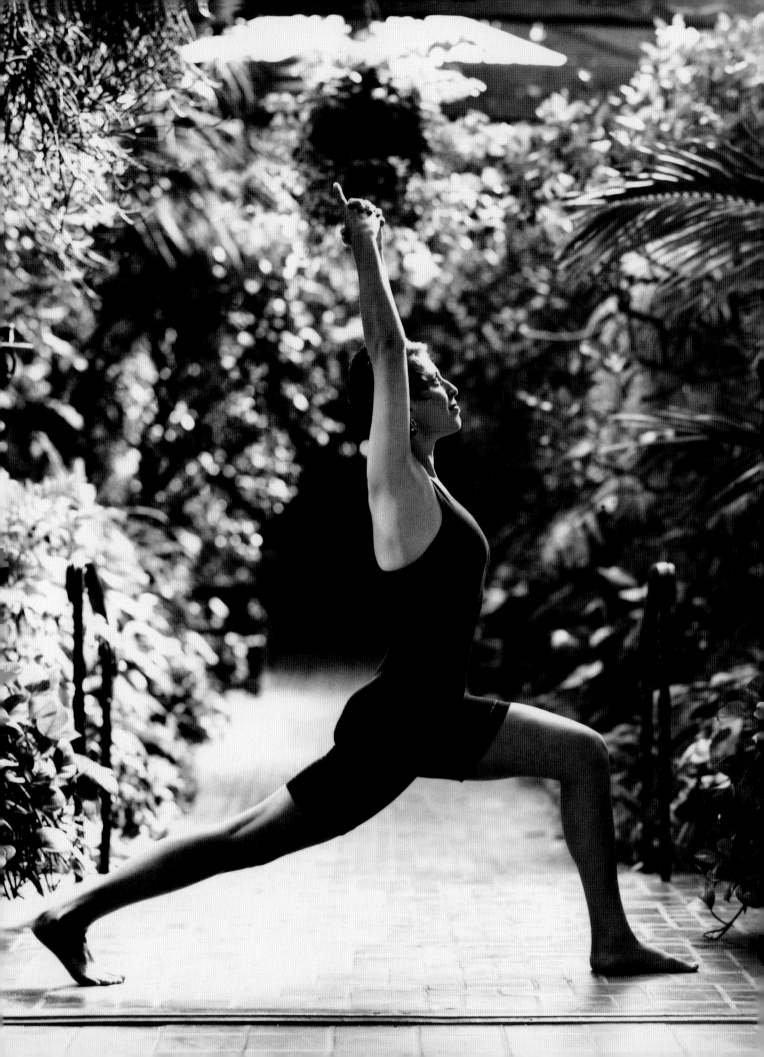

CONFIDENCE

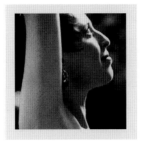

"You're lovable!" "You can do it!" "I trust you with this special secret." Affirmations like these are great Confidence builders. As children, we are ideally surrounded by adults who beam messages of approval and empowerment at us, helping to build the Spiritual Muscle of Confidence.

But too often all we hear as children are worries and warnings. Tell a child, "That's too hard for you," or "Be careful or you'll get hurt!" excessively, and the child grows up wary, fearful, and full of doubt. Early negative feedback can damage our self-esteem. We learn to believe that we are not good enough, that we do not deserve things in life, that we are not capable of learning difficult skills.

For many of us, our worst times at school were gym days (especially when the class was picking teams). We thought our competence was measured by how well we competed. If we were picked last or our team lost, we got the message we were losers.

As adults, the critical messages we heard as children often run in our heads over and over, like an audio tape on continuous play. We grow so accustomed to this background noise that we don't even realize it's on. However, we do have a choice. We can press the eject button and select a tape of self-affirming messages.

Integrating new, positive ideas takes time, but keep repeating these words of empowerment in whatever ways work for you: sing them, dance them, draw them, write them. Start each yoga session, for example, with the statement, "I am a highly skilled yoga practitioner!" Or, while holding a challenging pose, proclaim emphatically, "This posture is getting easier every day!" Repetition creates an internal memory structure that will help erase the old tapes.

In the meantime, act as if you *are* confident. Make *believe* that you *believe* in yourself! Cultivating competence does not mean becoming cocky, defensive, or egotistical. Rather, it is your birthright to feel assured of who you are. Our minds, for short periods of time, don't know the difference between real and imagined events; mark your determination for success in any endeavor, whether worldly or spiritual, with the adage that many spiritual masters have pronounced in different ways: "Fake it till you make it!"

The technique of pretending to a level of mastery higher than you have already achieved is part of many spiritual paths. Some Tibetan Buddhists practice each day imagining that they are already enlightened. Acting with conviction is easier if they make believe that they have already attained a more evolved level of spiritual development.

Our deepest fear is not that we are inadequate.

Our deepest fear is that we are powerful beyond measure.

It is our light, not our darkness, that most frightens us.

We ask ourselves, who am I to be brilliant, gorgeous, talented and fabulous?

Actually, who are you not to be?

You are a child of God. Your playing small doesn't serve the world.

There's nothing enlightened about shrinking so that other people won't feel insecure around you.

We are born to manifest the glory of God that is within us.

It's not just in some of us; it's in everyone.

And as we let our own light shine, we consciously give other people permission to do the same.

As we are liberated from our own fear, our presence automatically liberates others.

— MARIANNE WILLIAMSON, FROM *A RETURN TO LOVE*

You can use a similar skill to boost your Confidence in your yoga practice. Center yourself and see yourself in your mind's eye performing a posture effortlessly and with perfect form. Rehearsing skills on your inner practice mat will help you feel more powerful when you are actually moving your body.

In everyday activities, acting confident can get you over rough spots. Nearly everyone gets nervous before speaking in front of a group, for example. In some studies, fear of public speaking actually surpasses fear of death. The great Shakespearean actor Sir Laurence Olivier suffered from acute stage fright, though you'd never know it from watching him on the stage or screen.

Some of us are afraid we might actually succeed. Our previous efforts at boldness may have been met with jealousy, rejection, and isolation. Fear of success leads to self-sabotage, which undermines future achievements and past triumphs.

Confidence doesn't mean never experiencing fear. Like any other emotion, fear comes up, washes through us, and subsides. If we resist fear, however, it becomes locked in our bodies, constricting the breath, muscles, and even thought. Through conscious movement, we can transform the energy of fear into excitement and Confidence.

As you practice yoga, you will develop trust and faith in your body and its abilities. Yoga is 100 percent noncompetitive. You are not even competing with yourself. And there's no funny gym uniform!

A confident body leads to a confident mind. Stand tall, hold your head high atop a long spine. Take in a deep breath, bathing your divine inner self in confident energy. Gather a sense of assurance. Keep this sense with you even as your body vibrates, sweats, or shakes during your yoga practice. The trembling will allow your mind to release the grip of fear.

The Spiritual Muscle of Confidence will grow and blossom as the truth of who you are unfolds.

Postures for Confidence Standing Swings, Mountain, and Warrior I will flex your Confidence muscles. Triangle and Cobra continue to enhance your belief in yourself. You'll find there's nothing you can't do! When you create your own posture, you will draw upon the inherent Confidence of the Mountain to pave the way to finding your own symbolic pose of self-esteem.

Breathing Lesson for Confidence The Sun Breath brings steady assurance with each inhalation and exhalation.

Relaxation for Confidence Take yourself on an adventure where you discover how to "Transform Fear Into Excitement."

YOGA STORY FOR CONFIDENCE:
KRIS JACOBSEN

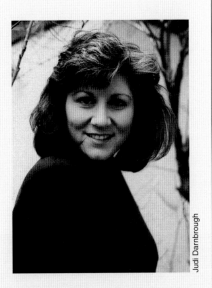

Judi Darnbrough

Until we change how we feel about ourselves, most efforts toward self-improvement fail. Kris Jacobsen had tried many different diets and weight loss programs. Then she signed up for a yoga class. Not only did she lose all of the extra weight, she also changed her whole lifestyle.

My weight has always been a constant battle. When I am anxious, I put on even more weight. I had a lot of self-doubt starting at a new school. I had been waiting to break up with my boyfriend of six years, but his emotional state was fragile—his brother was dying of cancer. Consciously or subconsciously, I hoped he would break up with me if I were heavy.

Before I started doing yoga, I didn't see the dynamic of a pattern I had repeated throughout my life. When I don't trust life, but instead wait (weight) for it to get better, I put on weight. Then I don't feel good about myself, so I eat some more. It's a vicious cycle.

I didn't know the solution would be as easy or as enjoyable as yoga.

My Confidence level started to rise when I mastered the Triangle. When I first tried it, I couldn't do it and breathe at the same time. I practiced outside of class twice a day, and within a month, I found it easier to breathe while holding the pose. I felt so accomplished and successful that I knew I was on the road to Confidence. When I'm in the Triangle, I look up as I stretch myself instead of looking down in a depressed and contracted way.

I became conscious of how I hold my breath when I am nervous, overwhelmed, or worried. I started to breathe through not only the Triangle, but also other difficulties in my life. I began to recognize that breathing through the things that make me anxious is where my power lies.

The vicious cycle began to reverse. I began to let go of the extra weight, and I stopped waiting for something outside of myself to magically help me. I lost thirty-three pounds, and what I gained is immeasurable. I tuned in to my body and fell in love with it. Practicing yoga is like taking a Confidence vitamin.

---

*Earth, Water, Fire, and Air / Within me all things are there / Flesh on my bones is like the Earth /
It's soft but strong and full of worth / The blood that flows within my veins /
Is like the ocean, river, and rain / My spirit soars and takes me higher / Here is where I keep my fire /
My breath and thoughts are like the air / I can do everything and go anywhere /
Earth, water, fire, and air / Within me all things are there / And so I pledge unto myself /
Power, love, health, and wealth*

—LUISA TEISH, FROM *JAMBALAYA*

STANDING SWINGS

Body Benefits:

➤ Rotates and aligns spine

➤ Strengthens spinal nerves

➤ Stimulates circulation of blood and oxygen to spine

➤ Energizes and heats body

Yoga Tip Have you ever watched a talented dancer? Though her arms and legs may be involved in such moves as high kicks or rapid twirls, the center of her body is grounded and confident. A door swings on its hinges time and time again while remaining fixed, solid and fully attached to the wall. Keep your torso upright and your knees soft. Let your arms flap like empty coat sleeves while maintaining an assured steadiness. Be loose and gentle with the movements. Confidence is not found in rigidity, but rather in free, relaxed motion.

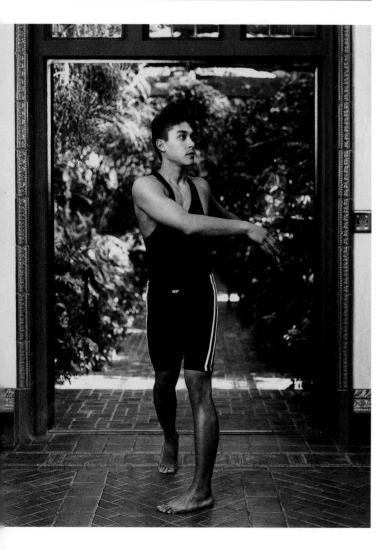

Let's begin:

1. Start from Proper Standing Alignment with your arms at your sides and your feet a little more than hip width apart.

2. Begin to twist the hips from side to side. When you twist to the right, look over the right shoulder and lift the left heel. When you twist to the left, look over the left shoulder and lift the right heel.

3. Allow the arms to follow the twisting movement. As they swing around the body, allow the flapping to create a steady rhythm.

4. Inhale through your nose when you face front, and exhale audibly through your mouth when you twist to either side.

5. Experiment with different speeds and paces of your movement and its coordinating breath.

6. Slow the movement down and eventually come back to stillness, standing with your arms at your sides.

7. Take a moment to pause and check in with how you are feeling.

To feel brave, act as if we were brave, use all of our will to that end, and a courage fit will very likely replace the fit of fear.

—WILLIAM JAMES

MOUNTAIN

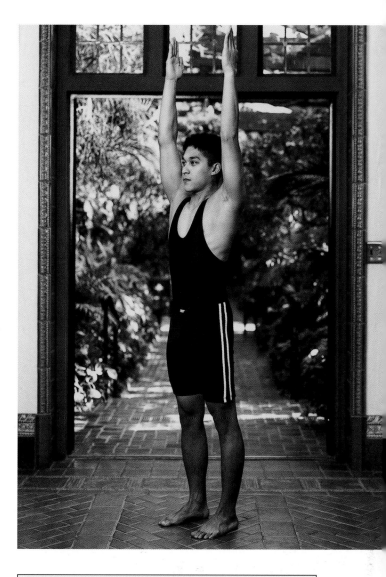

Body Benefits:

➤ Improves poor posture

➤ Strengthens ankles, knees, hips, back, neck, and shoulders

➤ Regulates functioning of kidneys

➤ Stimulates circulatory and respiratory systems

➤ Heats and invigorates entire system

➤ Creates stability and groundedness

Let's begin:

1. Begin in Proper Standing Alignment. Bring your fingers together and lengthen them straight toward the ground.

2. Extend your arms out to the sides. When they reach shoulder height, turn the palms up. Continue to lift the arms until they are directly overhead with the palms facing each other. You may hold them in a V position or parallel to each other, depending on which best suits your body.

3. Keep your elbows straight, shoulders relaxed.

4. Fix your gaze on a point on the wall ahead of you at eye level.

5. Take several deep, full breaths in this posture. Imagine yourself as a mountain grounded in the earth while reaching proudly toward the sky.

6. Release the posture by slowly lowering the arms straight out to shoulder height. At this point, turn the palms down and continue until your arms reach your sides.

7. Take a moment to stand with your eyes closed. Check in with yourself and notice any shifts in your attitude, energy, or emotions.

When to avoid this posture Do not hold for long periods of time if you are pregnant or have high blood pressure, a history of heart disease, or nervous disorders.

Yoga Tip This posture seems so basic that you may decide to pass over it. Actually, it is one of the most significant and beneficial postures you can ever learn. Without even realizing it, we sometimes stand in a way that contributes to physical and emotional discomfort. The Mountain posture is a powerful reminder of our inherent ability to stand on our own two feet.

It seems funny that something so simple can give you such a feeling of accomplishment.

BECKY BLAUVELT, YOGA STUDENT

SUN BREATH

Body Benefits:

➤ Invigorates body

➤ Improves circulation and respiration

➤ Clears mind

➤ Rids lungs of stale air

➤ Stimulates digestion

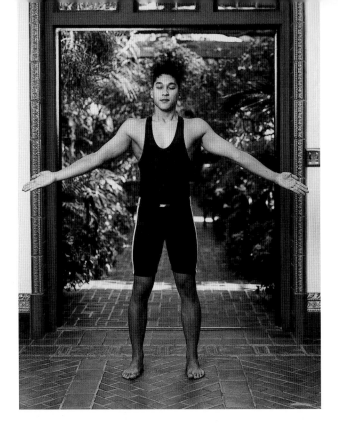

Let's begin:

1. Start in Proper Standing Alignment with your arms at your sides and your fingers together. You can practice the Sun Breath with eyes open or closed.

2. Inhale slowly through the nose and raise your arms with palms facing out to the sides and up overhead until the backs of the fingers meet. Synchronize your arm movements so that your hands meet as you complete the inhalation.

3. Exhale through the mouth with a sigh as you lower the arms back down to your sides, palms down. Move the arms with control as though you are pushing through water. Time your arm movements so that your hands come back to your sides as you complete the exhalation.

4. Repeat steps 2 and 3 several times. Make sure your shoulders stay relaxed even as you lift the arms.

5. To complete the exercise, lower the arms to your sides. Stand in stillness with your eyes closed and notice any shift in your energy.

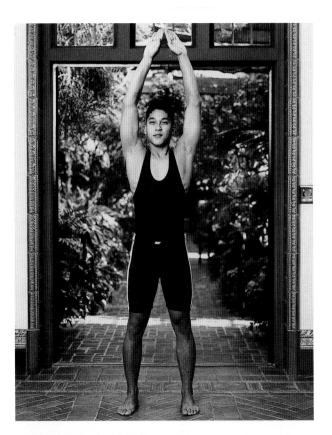

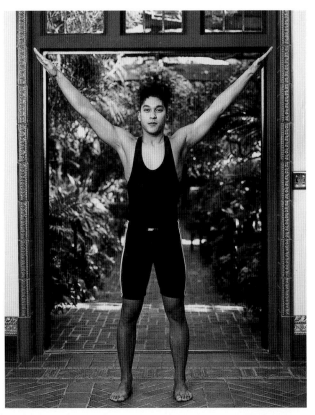

When to avoid this posture Do not practice for long periods of time if you are pregnant, if you have high blood pressure, a history of heart disease, or nervous disorders.

Yoga Tip If you start to feel lightheaded from all of the oxygen being drawn into your system, simply stop. Sit down and your breathing will return to normal. With practice, you will become more accustomed to the increase in oxygen. Build slowly. You wouldn't just put on your sneakers and run ten miles if you were out of shape, would you? Baby steps and breathing are the keys to building Confidence. The will to literally *breathe* through life's experiences can transform a tragedy into profound learning, fear into an opportunity to trust.

CREATE YOUR OWN POSTURE FOR CONFIDENCE

In this exercise, you will hold the Mountain posture that you learned earlier. Before you begin, determine your level of ability. If you are a beginner, hold for two or three minutes. Intermediate students can hold for three to five minutes or longer. Use a timer or have a clock available.

When to avoid this posture: For pregnant or menstruating women, or those with high blood pressure, history of heart disease or stroke, or weak knees, hold the Mountain for only a few breaths. Use the energy you build in that amount of time to bring you into a meditation in motion.

Let's begin:

1. Start in Proper Standing Alignment.

2. Move into the Mountain and readjust yourself so that you are in alignment.

3. Breathe down into your belly. Keep your eyes fixed on a point on the wall in front of you.

4. Hold for the amount of time that you determined before you started. As you hold the posture, use your breath to support you through difficult moments.

5. Notice all of the sensations that occur during this time of holding—what they feel like, where they are, and whether or not they move or change.

6. Let out any sounds that might want to come out: sighs, moans, groans.

7. Once you have held the Mountain for the time determined (or as close as you can come to it), close your eyes and begin to release the posture in *slow* motion.

8. Allow your mind to take a back seat as your body moves in whatever way it wants to. You may be surprised at what happens: your arms may remain suspended in midair, you might bend forward at the waist and hang, you may come into another yoga posture, or an infinite number of other movements.

9. As if you were in an unplanned, slow-motion dance, let your body continue moving, pausing, and exploring until it finds a position it wants to rest in.

10. Hold this position for as long as you wish. Receive the confident energy that comes from listening and trusting your body's wisdom.

11. When you feel complete, take the time to name your posture(s) and write down your experiences: your feelings, the movements you went in and out of, your thoughts, and anything else you feel is relevant. Know that as you develop the capacity to trust your body's wisdom, you will become more confident in your daily life.

TRIANGLE

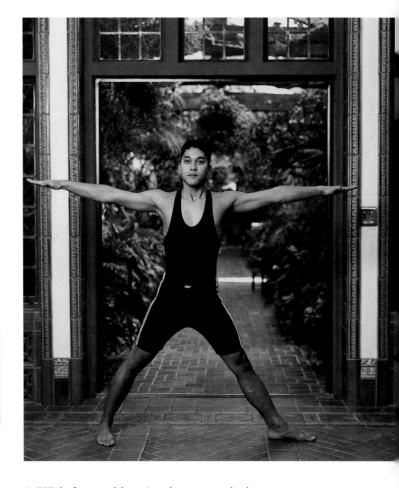

Body Benefits:

➤ Stretches and strengthens lateral, dorsal, and intercostal muscles

➤ Helps align and strengthen spine

➤ Strengthens feet, back, arms, neck, shoulders, and joints

➤ Aids digestion, respiration, and circulation

➤ Energizes and decongests nervous system

➤ Rejuvenates spinal nerves, veins, and tissues

➤ Increases flexibility in hips, ankles, and knees

➤ Great for menstrual discomforts and male reproductive disorders

Let's begin:

1. Start in Proper Standing Alignment. Place the feet a leg's length apart (about three feet).

2. Imagine that your hip bones are headlights on a car. Throughout this pose, keep both headlights facing front.

3. Lift your arms out to the sides in a T position. The palms face down (fingers together) and the elbows are straight.

4. Turn the left foot so that the toes point in the same direction as your left hand. Turn the right toes in so that they point slightly to the left. The left heel is in line with the right arch.

5. Keep the hips facing forward even though they will naturally want to turn.

Yoga is a pep talk you give yourself!

—AMY MARCUS, YOGA STUDENT

---

6. With feet and legs in place, stretch the torso to the left as you press the right hip away toward the right. Reach to the left with your left hand. Your head should be in line with your spine, tilting toward the left.

7. Reach to the left as far as you can. Once again, leave the feet and legs in place as you rotate only the arms. Lower the left arm down toward the left foot and extend the right arm overhead. Focus on spreading the hands away from each other in one straight line. Don't slouch in an effort to touch your fingertips to the ground. Your hand may rest anywhere along your leg as you gradually develop more flexibility.

8. If your neck is strong, turn the head to look at your right hand. If not, look forward or down.

9. Breathe into the stretch created along the right side of the body. Elongate and feel the sensations as the body opens up to receive more air.

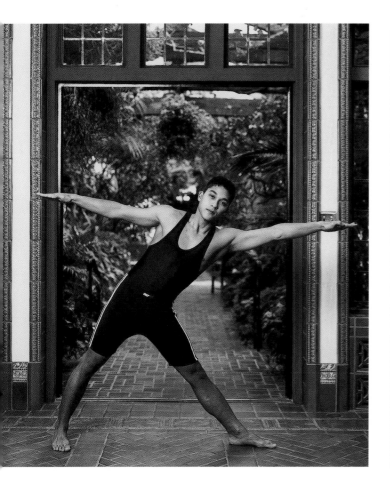

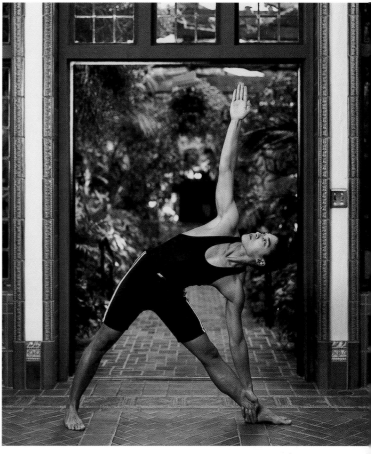

10. Imagine that your body is between two panes of glass so that it stays in one plane. Keep the legs active and strong.

11. To release, bring the right arm up and to the right as if someone is reaching out a hand to help you. This will return you to standing position with your arms outstretched in a T.

12. Keep your arms extended out to the sides as you shift your foot positions to practice the Triangle on the opposite side. If you need a break, lower the arms. Repeat steps 3–9 to the right side.

13. When you have done the Triangle on both sides, lower the arms and bring the feet back underneath your hips.

14. Close your eyes for a moment and stand in stillness. Check in and notice how the body feels. Become aware of the quality of your breath.

When to avoid this posture Do not hold for long periods of time if you are pregnant or menstruating, if you have high blood pressure, or if you have a history of heart disease, nervous disorders, or weak back muscles.

Yoga Tip Your ability to do the Triangle will vary from day to day. Some days you will find it more difficult than others. Before you do this pose, close your eyes and visualize yourself doing it with grace and ease. On the days when you would prefer to remain within your comfort zone, doing the Triangle anyway will boost your self-esteem. Meeting *this* challenge will help you to develop the Confidence needed to meet life's other challenges.

COBRA

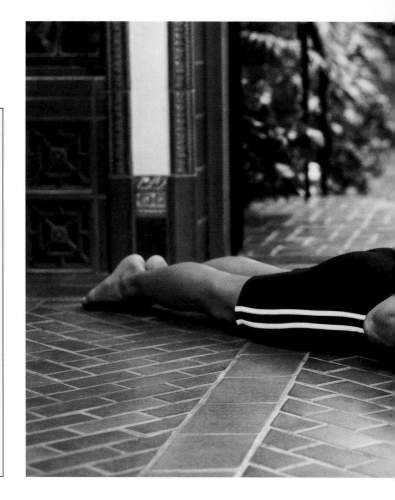

Body Benefits:

➤ Heats and invigorates body

➤ Opens lungs and expands rib cage and chest

➤ Delivers fresh blood and oxygen to pelvis and reproductive organs

➤ Rejuvenates kidneys

➤ Improves digestive functioning and relieves constipation

➤ Relieves menstrual and menopausal discomfort

➤ Strengthens arm, shoulder, wrist, and back muscles

➤ Tones, aligns, strengthens, and flexes spine

➤ Relaxes nervous system

Let's begin:

1. Lie on your belly. Rest your forehead on the floor. Spread your fingers apart and place your hands underneath your shoulders with your elbows as close to the body as possible.

2. Draw the legs together. Imagine that you can zip them up from toes to buttocks. If this is too difficult, leave the legs slightly apart. Keep the buttocks squeezed and press the pelvic triangle (the two hip bones and the pubic bone) down into the floor.

3. Wiggle your torso out of the waist. Keep the shoulders relaxed and press the crown of the head away from the feet.

4. Using the strength of your back, lift the upper body beginning with the forehead, nose, chin, and finally neck, shoulders, and upper chest. You can even lift your hands off the floor for a second to ensure that your back muscles are doing the work. (Look Ma, no hands!)

5. Return your palms to the floor. Press down into your hands, lifting the middle torso off the ground. Be aware of your shoulders riding up toward the ears. Draw them down through the back. Keep the elbows bent and close to the body.

6. Fix your gaze on a point on the wall at or above eye level. Maintain open and deep breathing. Hold until you reach your toleration level.

7. When you are ready to release, keep the buttocks squeezed tight and begin to roll back down from the middle belly all the way to the forehead.

If you have no enthusiasm, put on a front. Act enthusiastic and the feeling will become genuine.

— RABBI NACHMAN OF BRATSLAV

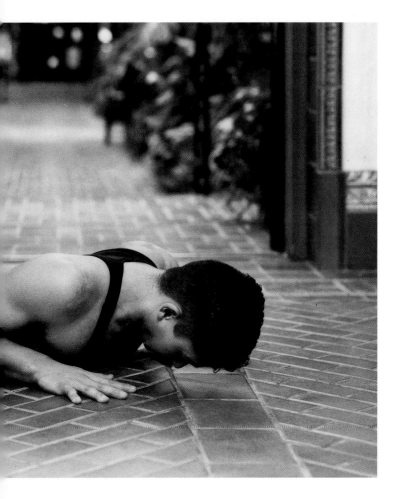

When to avoid this posture Do not practice the Cobra after the third month of pregnancy. If you have suffered recent abdominal surgery or abdominal inflammation, avoid the Cobra.

Yoga Tip The only thing we can count on is change. We need Confidence to face the changes in our lives. The Cobra is a symbol of regeneration and rebirth. Images of snakes are found in many ancient temples around the world. Practicing this posture offers you a visceral experience of opening to change. You shed your old skin and come into the next season of your life with greater self-trust when you become the Cobra time and time again.

8. Once you have come back to the original position, turn the head to one side, close your eyes, release the buttocks, and rest. You may want to windshield-wipe the lower legs from side to side or in and out (in either the American or the European version).

9. To counterbalance the back bending, fold your hips back to your heels into the Child Pose.

WARRIOR I

Body Benefits:

➤ Stimulates circulatory and respiratory systems

➤ Stretches and firms inner thigh muscles

➤ Energizes and decongests nervous system

➤ Improves digestion

➤ Strengthens legs, hip joints, arms, shoulders, and neck

➤ Helps align the spine

➤ Heats and invigorates body

When to avoid this posture Do not hold for long periods of time if you are pregnant, have high blood pressure, or have a history of heart disease or nervous disorders.

Yoga Tip Do not place the moving foot *in line* with the stationary foot, as on a tightrope or balance beam, or you will lose your stability. To maintain balance in this posture, step directly forward as if you were a warrior taking a giant step toward victory.

Let's begin:

1. Start in Proper Standing Alignment.

2. As you inhale, draw your arms up overhead into the Mountain.

3. Exhale through your mouth as you bring the right foot forward several feet in front of you with the right knee bent. Keep the right foot flat on the floor even though the left heel is off the ground.

4. Be sure to keep the left hip facing forward and the right knee directly over the right ankle.

5. Breathe full deep breaths into this powerful posture. Press the fingertips up toward the ceiling.

6. To release, step forward or backward to the original starting position. Stepping backward is more challenging.

7. Repeat steps 1–6 on the opposite side.

8. Once you have completed both sides, stand with the eyes closed and notice how you feel.

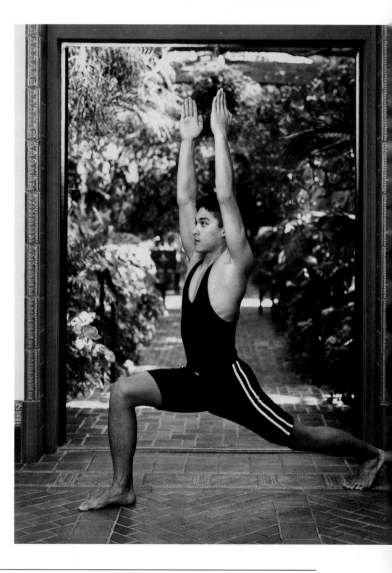

There's no showing off to see who can do the 'best yoga.'... There is only a push to learn the most about yourself.

—KATHY BLEVINS, YOGA STUDENT

TRANSFORMING FEAR INTO EXCITEMENT

1. Come into your favorite variation of the Corpse Pose.

2. Take several long, deep breaths. Slow down your mind's pace by slowing down the rhythm of your breath. Continue to regulate your breathing for two or three minutes.

3. Call to mind a situation that causes you fear or anxiety. It could be chronic or more specific.

4. Replay this scene in your mind's eye as if you were watching it on the movie screen inside your head.

5. As you quiet your mind, contact the place inside your body where the fear resides. We often hold fear in a certain part of the body. It can manifest as any sensation including tightness, soreness, heaviness, emptiness, pain, heat, cold, or tingling.

6. Feel the sensations. Know that you are perfectly safe at this moment and trust that the fear is actually a friend in disguise.

7. As if you were an observer, notice the details of the fear sensation. Does it have a color? If so, what color? What is the texture of the sensation? The shape? You may feel as though you are making it up. Know that all of the information you receive comes from you—from your body, mind, and various levels of consciousness. Allow yourself the luxury of going *with* it instead of resisting it.

8. Notice how much energy these sensations carry within them. Fear is loaded with strength and power. Instead of cutting off from these feelings, embrace them with your breath.

9. Notice how this "fear" has the same quality of energy and heightened alertness as "excitement."

10. Now shift gears for a moment. Imagine now that you could rise or fly up above your body and look down on it. See it resting on the floor from a bird's eye view.

11. As you observe yourself, imagine that you could see your body lying next to a door. Notice what the door looks like—its shape, color, size, what it's made of.

12. On the other side of the door is a place where transformation takes place. Now see yourself getting up and moving through this doorway.

13. Once you cross the threshold, recall the situation that brought up the anxiety. See yourself doing the very thing that you fear, handling it with the help of all of the energy that was trapped in your body. Allow the energy of fear to become enthusiasm. Feel your fear transforming into excitement, power, and deep inner faith.

14. Watch the fear transform: see the colors change, the texture alter, and the shapes move. With fear as an ally named excitement, we can experience more of our potential.

15. As you unleash this sense of vitality, breathe into it and allow it to wash over you. Feel your bodymind as limitless and notice the comfort this sense brings. Enjoy this feeling as long as you wish. When you feel complete, feel your body once again lying on the floor.

16. Begin to deepen your breath. In your own time, roll over onto one side with your knees curled in towards your chest. Transition slowly into a comfortable seated position. Remain with your eyes closed experiencing a state of freshness, alertness, and a sense of balanced excitement.

Whatever you can do, or dream you can, begin it. Boldness has genius, power and magic in it.

GOETHE

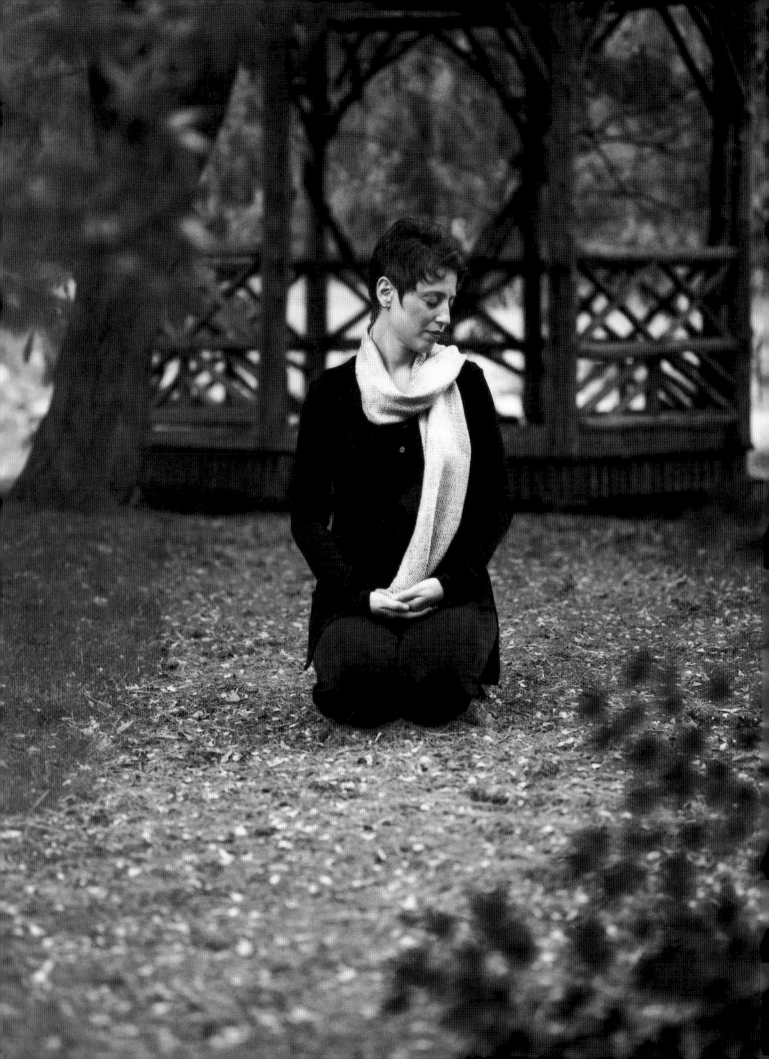

PEACE

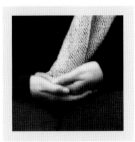

Siblings rival, nations battle, even lawn mowers and leaf blowers disturb the Peace.

How is it possible to develop inner Peace in a world where disorder and hostility abound?

Imagine that everyone in the world dropped what they were doing right now, came

outside their homes and workplaces, and sat in an enormous circle that spiraled around

the earth. Visualize the Peace pipe being passed to every being across enemy lines, from one

race and ethnic group to another, from one family member to another. To carry this image

within your consciousness is to affirm that Peace can exist.

Before we can bring Peace into our communities, we must first develop it inside ourselves. We can experience both a visceral tranquillity in the body and cultivate mental calm through the practice of yoga. Stilling the turbulent waters of the mind helps anchor the body.

Picture yourself at an amusement park. Imagine you can put only your mind and all of its thoughts on the ride. Now that you are unattached to them, you can watch them as they move up and down and as they go through their many twists and turns.

The mind is a funny thing; sometimes when it's being watched, it gets embarrassed at the crazy things it's thinking. Once you observe your thoughts and discover what they are, you begin to realize that they are just that, *thoughts*. They run the gamut from pleasant to disturbing, frightening to amusing, loving to destructive, logical to absurd.

You may notice that you hold onto certain

thoughts whether they serve you or not. Most of us think the same thoughts we were thinking yesterday, which will also be tomorrow's thoughts. Observe your thoughts as if they were clouds floating along in the sky. Clouds, like thoughts, come and go. Once we are liberated from the chains of our thoughts, we are left with what has always been there, our ever available companion, Peace.

But don't wait for picture-perfect moments of serenity, like meditating on a secluded mountain top, to bring Peace into your daily life. Remind yourself that a traffic jam is better than a traffic accident. Hum to yourself during thunder storms. Cultivate a peaceful heart by forgiving those who have been unkind. Let your inner tranquillity reverberate out to all beings.

Prayers for Peace are a part of nearly every cultural tradition in the world. More than a thousand years ago, a Native American wise man known as the Peacemaker gave to his people the Great Law of Peace. His Thanksgiving Address, a petition for the blessing of Peace on all living things, is still spoken by the Native Iroquois (or Six Nations: the Mohawk, Oneida, Cayuga, Onondaga, Seneca, and Tuscarora) of upstate New York and Canada at the beginning and ending of formal meetings. Whoever speaks the prayers does so in their own words.

Use your own inner (or outer) voice to open and close each yoga session. Invoke the spirit of calm and serenity to smooth out the wrinkles of conflict and discord. Let your movements and stillness be guided by the peacemaker inside you. Your body will respond immediately to this kinesthetic quieting.

You may also allow a few moments of complete quiet before or after your yoga practice or in between each posture. Protect silence as you would an endangered species. It is within the rests or spaces between notes that beautiful music is created. The innermost secrets of a dear friend are whispered or unspoken. The sacred essence of dance is captured in a performer's body when it is still or momentarily suspended.

As you cultivate inner serenity, you can ease a quickened pulse, slow a rapid heart rate, and relax muscles. Moving slowly and savoring every sensuous micromovement will help you call a truce to internal bickering. By bringing harmony to the mind through such absorption, your body is serenaded with a soothing hymn. Hold a pose with reverence and experience the grace of the posture. Let each movement be a prayer that you offer as a covenant for Peace.

Postures for Peace Neck Rolls, Seated Yoga Mudra, and the Hero will help you create a powerful peacetime. The Half-Shoulderstand will give you a whole new perspective on the definition of calm, while the Seated Forward Bend ends the formal session as you turn your focus to the quiet place within.

Breathing Lesson for Peace There's No Place Like Home is an opportunity to chant the healing vibration of "home."

Meditation for Peace Inner Sanctuary helps you create your own sacred place that you can visit time and again.

NECK OPENERS

> **Body Benefits:**
> ➤ Increases flexibility and strength in neck
> ➤ Helps regulate thyroid function
> ➤ Lubricates neck joints
> ➤ Relieves neck and shoulder tension
> ➤ Firms chin

Let's begin:

Part I

1. Come into Proper Sitting Alignment with eyes open or closed.

2. Slowly lower your chin to your chest, moving only the head. Keep your torso erect.

3. With your chin close to the chest, slide your chin up toward the right shoulder so that if your eyes are open, you'll be looking over your right shoulder.

4. Hold and breathe deeply for several breaths into the opening created on the left side of the neck.

5. Slide the chin back down to the center of the chest, and then continue on to bring it up toward the left shoulder. Again, hold and breathe into the opening created on the right side of the neck.

6. Slowly slide the chin back to center and repeat this half circle two more times before you lift the head back into an upright position.

7. Now lift the chin toward the ceiling (not shown). Do not release the weight of the head by throwing it back. Instead, extend the chin up while maintaining a straight spine.

8. You may find some sounds or yawns that want to be released. Let them out.

9. Now imagine that you are chewing a piece of gum. Focus on stretching the throat and jaw as you chew.

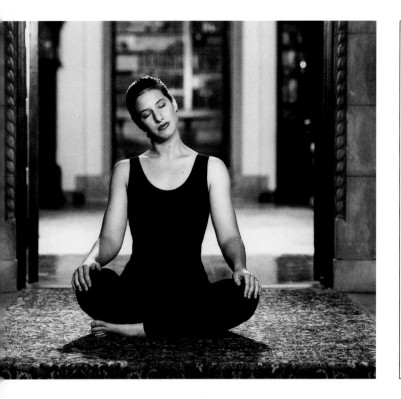

Yoga Tip The neck plays a significant role in our emotional life. Try communicating with this part of the body and listen for the kinesthetic feeling. The neck is the physical bridge between the body and the mind. For messages to be sent from one part to the other, they must move through the neck's "post office." Often news gets tied up here and stays stuck in the neck as tension, tightness, or even severe spasm. What the body feels and the mind thinks can get tied up in the neck, and the neck may not know how to process the information. Opening up the neck is like sending a relief crew to the main post office during the holiday rush.

10. Close the mouth, slowly bring your head back to its natural upright position. Pause and notice how you are carrying your head at this moment.

In yoga, there's no pressure to get this or that right; it's a carefree period of "down time."

—DAWN OWENS, YOGA STUDENT

Part II

11. Lengthen your spine once again. Drop the left ear toward the left shoulder. Keep the right shoulder down and relaxed. First simply allow the weight of your head to open up the right side of the neck.

12. Lift the left arm up and overhead. Place your left hand on the right ear. Without pulling on the ear, simply use the hand to encourage the neck to release.

13. Breathe fully into the stretch.

14. Release the left hand from your ear and return it to your knee. Allow the head to float back up to center. Notice the difference between the left and the right side of the neck.

15. Repeat steps 11–14 on the opposite side.

16. When you have completed both sides, sit in silence for a moment and notice the shift in your internal experience.

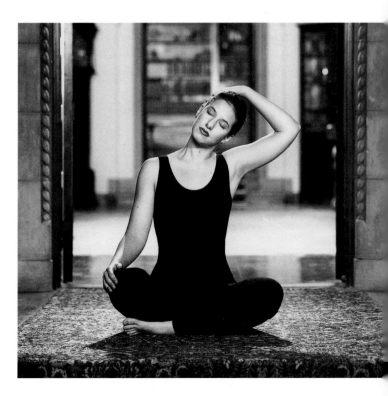

HERO

Body Benefits:

➤ Opens hips and legs

➤ Stretches spinal column

➤ Invigorates nervous system

➤ Stimulates peristalsis (digestive action)

➤ Stimulates kidneys, liver, gall bladder, and spleen

➤ Frees shoulders and neck from stiffness

When to avoid this posture Do not practice the Hero after the third month of pregnancy.

Yoga Tip Use essential oils during your yoga practice to establish a fragrant sanctuary of Peace. Lavender and geranium can help you deal with physical, mental, and chemical stress (pollutants) and are safe for everyone, including pregnant women. These aromatic oils are natural sedatives, antidepressants, and contain antiseptic properties.

They can be used before an exam or presentation to relax you, or before going to bed for a restful sleep. Important: do not use essential oils directly on the skin or internally. They are highly concentrated and potent. One or two drops of *pure* essential oil are all you need.

Every night in sleep you have a taste of peace and joy. While you are in deep slumber, God makes you live in the tranquil superconsciousness, in which all the fears and worries of this existence are forgotten. By meditation you can experience that holy state of mind when you are awake, and be constantly immersed in healing peace.

—PARAMAHANSA YOGANANDA

Let's begin:

1. Come into a seated position on your sitting bones with your legs bent in front of you and your feet on the ground.

2. Slide your left foot under the right leg with your left ankle resting on the ground. Bring the left foot as close to the right hip as possible.

3. Cross your right leg over the left by bending the knee. Most of us have tight hips, so bring the right leg only as far as you comfortably can. Eventually you will be able to line up your knees one atop the other.

4. To facilitate this leg position, place your hands in

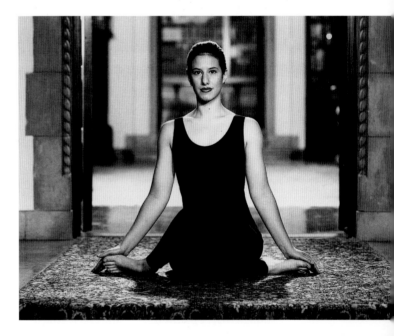

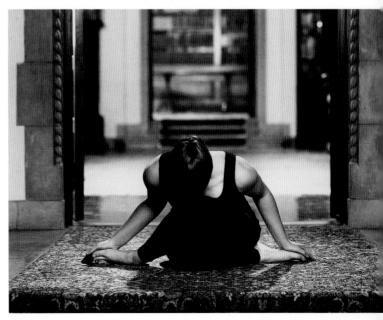

YOGA STORY FOR PEACE: BERNICE LEWIS

We all have hectic, fast-paced lives. Bernice Lewis is a folk singer who at one point was driving solo thirty thousand miles a year in order to perform. Often without the comforts of home or a regular schedule, Bernice finds Peace in practicing yoga daily.

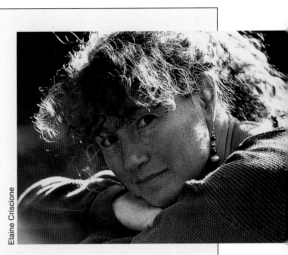

Elaine Criscione

See America from her guest rooms. As I travel from gig to gig, I stay in people's homes rather than paying for hotels. I'm often in a strange bed, the room is either too hot or too cold, and sometimes the sheets aren't clean. I once did yoga in a trailer in the eighteen-inch space that led up to the bed. I'm very protective of that sacred, quiet morning time because I'm such a blabbermouth the rest of the day. Yoga is invaluable in my line of work.

I spend most of the day traveling to gigs by car or plane. I'd probably have arthritis if didn't do yoga, because I sit *a lot*. I warm up with Neck Rolls because I have problems in my left shoulder and neck from playing guitar. I am practically addicted to forward bends—they bring me right to my core. The act of moving forward brings me into a place of hope.

Even when I'm in a strange home, I wake up early and practice yoga alone. Most everything I do is with an audience. Yoga gives me the chance to *not* have to be a performer. It's my break from talking or thinking or singing. I move through the postures in silent meditation. Yoga has helped me build a peaceful place inside myself. It is there that I practice forgiveness and connect to my inside world. I wouldn't be able to withstand the pressures of entertaining without it.

The principles of yoga and its benefits come in handy whether I'm doing a gig or leading singing workshops. I couldn't teach people to sing, to find their voices, without my background in yoga.

I can't imagine how people who *don't* do yoga feel inside their bodies. Sometimes I have to fight to get myself on the yoga mat, but it's worth it in terms of Peace of mind and Peace in my relationships. My friend, singer Rod McDonald, wrote "Stop the war within yourself and you won't need to fight with anyone else." That says it all.

front of you and lean forward, balancing on your knees. Then place your sitting bones back down and notice how your legs fold nicely.

5. Place your hands on the soles of your feet and lengthen the spine.

6. With a flat back, begin to draw the torso down over the bent legs in slow motion. Stop and pause every inch or so and take a few breaths.

7. When you come to the point where you can go no further, round your spine resting your chin on your chest.

8. Try to relax by sending your breath into the areas that hold the most tension and tightness. Back off the stretch if necessary to enable you to hold the pose for five to seven breaths.

9. To come out of the posture, press down into the sitting bones and roll up the spine, stacking the vertebrae one on top of the other.

10. Slowly unravel the legs using your hands to guide them into the opposite position (left leg over right).

11. Repeat steps 2–9 on the other side.

12. When you have completed both sides, come back into a comfortable seated position and close your eyes. Notice the effects of the Hero.

SEATED YOGA MUDRA

Body Benefits:

➤ Provides brain with fresh blood supply

➤ Activates kidney functioning

➤ Helps develop flexibility in arms, shoulders, hips, and legs

➤ Tones and stretches spinal column

➤ Stimulates digestion

➤ Stimulates pituitary and thyroid glands

➤ Strengthens muscles and nerves in abdomen and pelvis

When you close your eyes at night
And you dream that journey home
To the land where the lame walk
And the blind still see
Do you cross that Isle of Spirit with me?

— BERNICE LEWIS, CHORUS TO "ISLE OF SPIRIT" (FROM "THERE'S NO PLACE LIKE HOME")

When to avoid this posture Do not do Seated Yoga Mudra if you suffer from glaucoma, detached retina, or weak eye capillaries. It is not to be done if you have unmedicated high blood pressure, recent or chronic injury to or inflammation in shoulders or abdomen.

Yoga Tip Use the triggers that usually cause you to be jangled and stressed (such as an alarm clock, a ringing telephone, or a red light) as opportunities to apply a calming and peaceful technique. At Plum Village in France, Zen master and Peace advocate Thich Nhat Hahn rings a bell to remind people to take deep breaths and smile. Take a moment to breathe and smile before you do each pose.

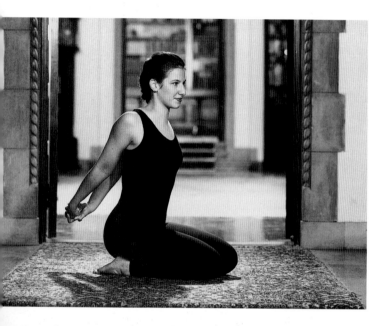

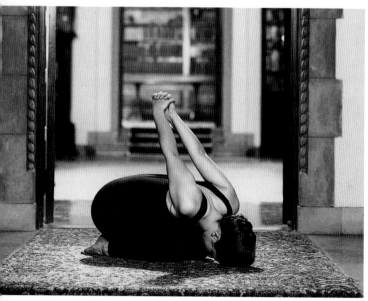

Let's begin:

1. Come into a kneeling position sitting on your heels. If this is uncomfortable, place a pillow beneath your buttocks.

2. Lift up through the spine and draw your attention to a calm, steady breathing pattern.

3. Lift your arms up in front of you with your palms facing away from each other. Then bring your hands behind you until they meet at the base of your spine.

4. Interlace your fingers. Squeeze the shoulder blades together, pressing the palms into each other.

5. On an exhalation, bring the torso forward from the hips with a flat back, until the forehead

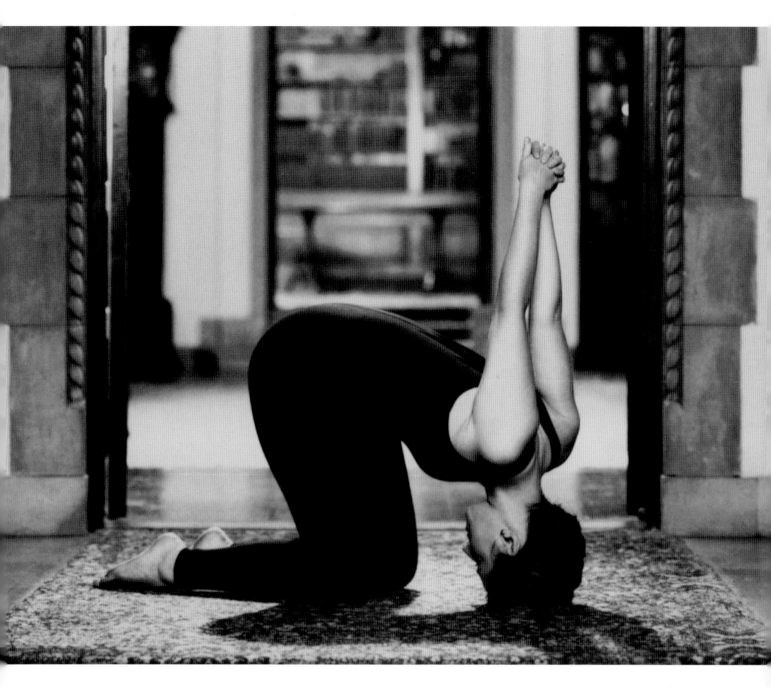

touches the floor. If this is too challenging, place a pillow on the floor so that you can rest your forehead on it. Keep the fingers interlaced even though the palms may have separated.

6. Take a few full, deep breaths here. If you feel challenged at this point, remain here.

7. For those of you who can proceed, lift the hips and roll up onto the crown of your head. Keep the majority of the weight on your shins.

8. Keep the breath flowing smoothly in this inverted position.

9. To release, slowly roll the forehead back down to the ground, lowering the hips.

10. Using the clasped hands to guide you, roll up the spine, stacking your vertebrae one on top of the other.

11. Once you are back in an upright kneeling position, slowly separate your hands and allow them to float back around in front of you, as if you are in a slow motion movie.

12. Sit in stillness for a moment and allow your body to recenter itself.

HALF-SHOULDERSTAND

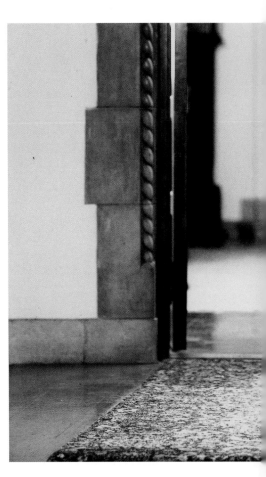

Body Benefits:

➤ Stimulates abdominal organs

➤ Improves facial complexion, scalp, and hair

➤ Enhances circulation and rests heart

➤ Counteracts gravity by allowing blood to flow to brain and upper body

➤ Stimulates thyroid and parathyroid

➤ Reduces muscular tension in neck and shoulders

➤ Rejuvenates system and relieves fatigue

➤ Helps prevent and relieve varicose veins and hemorrhoids

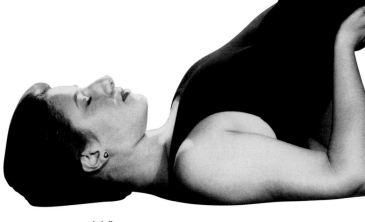

Before I learned yoga, I didn't know how to relax myself when I got upset, angry, or nervous. Yoga provided me with the tools.

—JENNIFER LESSER, YOGA STUDENT

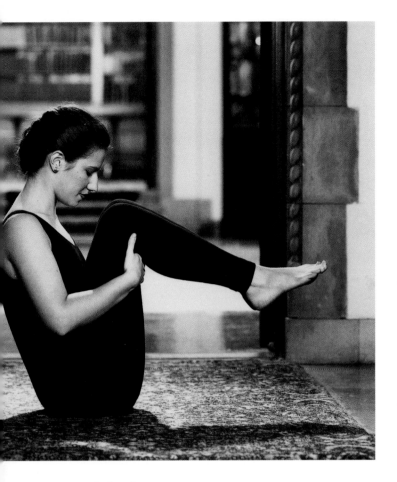

Let's begin:

1. Sit on your buttocks with your knees bent and held in close to your torso. Tuck your chin into your chest.

2. Roll back onto your spine. Lift and press the hips and legs up overhead. Keep your hands underneath your hips to support them. (If it is more comfortable, simply rest on your back and push your hips up overhead.)

3. Walk your shoulders together to create a padding for your neck or place a folded blanket or towel beneath your shoulders. If you have *any* discomfort in your neck at all, come out of the posture immediately.

4. Straighten your legs and allow the hips to rest into the support of your hands beneath them. The legs are not directly overhead. The weight of your pelvis is resting in your hands and arms.

5. Flex the feet toward you and keep the intention of a lengthened spine.

6. Find ways to relax deeply here. Let this be a posture of silence and stillness.

7. Remain in this position for as long as you comfortably can, between three and twenty breaths.

8. To release, walk your shoulder blades apart slightly and roll down onto your back.

9. Assume the Corpse Pose with your eyes closed. Feel the effects of this inverted posture.

When to avoid this posture Do not do the Half-Shoulderstand if you suffer from glaucoma, detached retina, or weak eye capillaries. Those with unmedicated high or low blood pressure should avoid this pose, as well as people with thyroid and chronic cervical (neck) or shoulder problems.

To keep your weight off the neck, place a folded towel or blanket underneath the shoulders and upper back. If this pose is too challenging, try the Legs-Up-The-Wall Corpse.

Yoga Tip Your attention will naturally go inward in this pose. Reversing gravity not only gives your internal organs a minivacation, but also allows your mind to look at the world from a different point of view. Give your body and your mind a break as you turn your perspective upside down.

SEATED FORWARD BEND

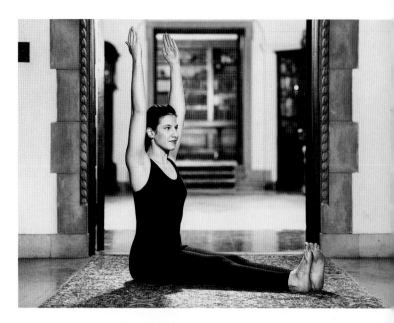

Body Benefits:

➤ Massages abdominal organs

➤ Lengthens, tones, and flexes spine

➤ Relieves constipation and promotes digestion

➤ Tones kidneys

➤ Supplies reproductive organs with fresh blood

➤ Stimulates nervous system

When to avoid this posture Practice carefully if you have sciatica. Separate the legs if you are pregnant and avoid pressure on the belly.

Yoga Tip Forward bends draw you into meditative stillness. This pose encourages a deep stretching of the backs of the legs. According to author/psychologist Ken Dychtwald, the hamstring muscles are related to control (self-control as well as being controlled), and when tight, often indicate difficulty in letting go. Use this posture to encourage letting go of issues that cause you to struggle: your image, tension, perfectionism, and need to control everything. As you shed these internal restraints, you will flow with life more easily.

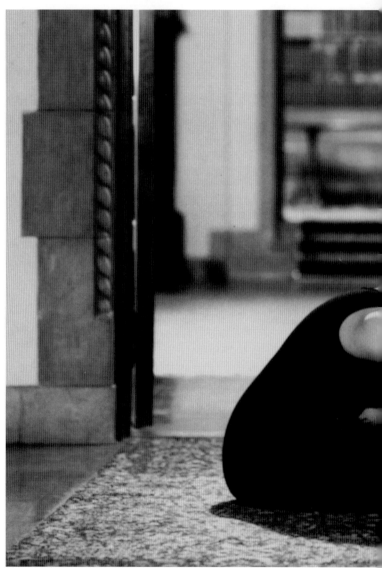

Let's begin:

1. Come into a seated position. Rock side to side with your legs outstretched in front of you. Come to rest on your sitting bones. Flex your toes back toward your face.

2. Breathe into a long, tall spine.

3. Raise your arms overhead beside your ears, palms facing each other. Keep the elbows straight.

4. With a flat back, begin to hinge at the hips, slowly extending the torso forward over your

legs. Keep your head in line with your spine and come forward a few inches at a time. Pause and breathe at each stopping point.

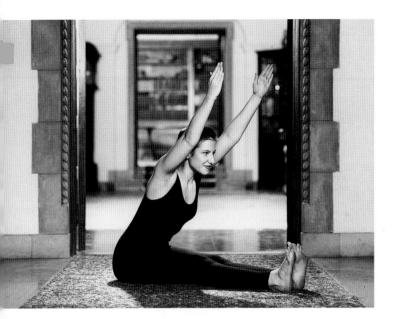

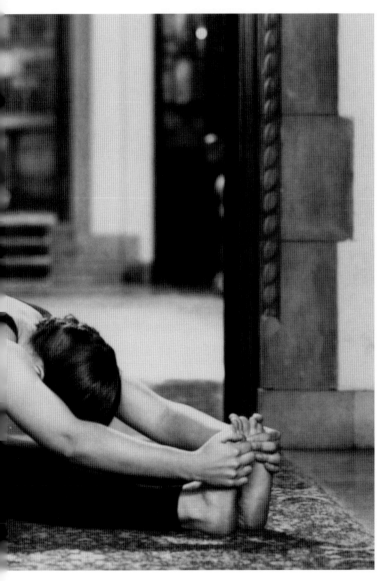

6. When you have extended the torso to the point of challenge (but not strain), drop the chin to the chest. Lower the arms and hands down to rest on the legs or feet.

7. Remain here, breathing comfortably for several breaths. If you can, hold in this dynamic yet peaceful pose for up to ten breaths.

8. To release, simply roll back up the spine, stacking the vertebrae one on top of the other, sliding your hands up your legs as you go.

9. Sit with your eyes closed and breathe out with a sigh.

5. If possible, keep the knees straight by pressing the heels away from you. Do bend them if you feel strain in your lower back or legs.

THERE'S NO PLACE LIKE HOME

Yoga Tip Have you ever noticed how good you feel after listening to your favorite song or singing in the shower? Sound is universally used for healing and releasing stress and is a simple and pleasurable way to remind us of our essence. The sound that is created in this exercise is similar to the Sanskrit sound, "Om," an ancient vibration known as the "sound of all sounds." Many traditions have similar prayerful sounds, such as the Judeo-Christian "Amen" or the Sufi "Amin." Benedictine monks chant from four to six hours a day, which helps them to maintain peaceful vitality. Yoga, breathing, relaxation, and meditation are all ways of coming home to the place where the true you resides.

1. Come into Proper Sitting Alignment with eyes closed. Allow your spine to be long and naturally erect.

2. Take several full, deep, long breaths.

3. Inhale through your nose and exhale with an audible sigh, singing or saying, "Hooooh," on a single note until you are comfortably out of air. Repeat this several times. Allow yourself to become absorbed in the sound as you feel it resonate in your belly and vibrate in your heart.

4. Now inhale, then exhale, sighing "Mmmm," on the same note, mouth closed. Repeat several times. Allow this vibration to resonate in your head.

5. Next, inhale through the nose. Combine the two sounds on the next exhalation with an open mouth, saying "Hoooh" and then "Mmmm" with a closed mouth. Feel your spine vibrate with this healing and soothing sound.

6. Practice this combination several times. Then simply sit in silence and listen to the sound of "home" as if it were an echo singing back to you. Feel the effects of sound vibration on your body and mind.

INNER SANCTUARY

Yoga Tip Musicologists and music therapists around the world use the works of Mozart, Bach, Beethoven, and other great composers to induce states of emotional, mental, and physical calm. Play soothing music for this experience (or any of the yoga postures for Peace). Let the harmony of the music wash over your body as you cultivate what mystics call a "still center." Let your internal tranquillity reverberate with universal Peace.

Let's begin:

1. Come into your favorite version of the Corpse Pose.

2. Take several long, deep, full breaths. Take a few minutes to rest and simply be in silence before you go on your peaceful journey.

3. Call to mind a special place that evokes a feeling of deep Peace, safety, and total relaxation. It may be a place that you have actually visited or one that exists in your imagination. Possible examples include the beach, the mountains, your bedroom or backyard, a European castle from a photo in a coffee-table book, your grandparents' farm.

4. With childlike imagination, as if you were watching a movie in your mind, picture this place with as much detail as possible. See the colors, textures, and shapes. Allow it to be exactly as you want it.

I happen to be of the belief that we would all be significantly better off if we spent more time getting acquainted with nothing.

—ED O'CONNOR,
YOGA STUDENT

114

5. Look around and notice if you are alone or if anyone else is there. Invite only those you want to be present.

6. Take note of the weather. If it isn't how you want, change it. Let the temperature be just perfect. Notice the quality of light. What time of day (or night) is it?

7. Take a deep breath and smell any aromas that surround you (ocean air, flowers, pine trees). If you cannot smell anything, that's OK too.

8. Listen carefully to hear any sounds, such as birds singing, wind blowing, or water flowing. You may simply hear the sound of silence.

9. Notice how you feel in this magical place that is your very own: safe, content, loved, serene, joyous. Imagine that you can breathe these feelings right into the core of your being, drawing them deeper and deeper within.

10. Take a moment to look around and see if you can find a small object. It could be a shell, a flower, a pine cone, or anything that calls to you.

11. Pick it up and hold it in your hand, knowing that your object represents this peaceful place. Look at it very carefully and then wait to see if it has a message for you. It can come to you in any form: sound, intuitive feeling, or written words, for example. Be patient and receptive. The message may come now or later.

12. If you are able to communicate with the object, you may wish to ask it for guidance on any issue in your life.

13. Once you feel complete, place this object in your pocket. If you received a message, repeat it to yourself.

14. Know that this place is always available to you and that you can return here whenever you wish.

15. Take one final look around, smell the scents, hear the sounds. Begin to deepen your breath, taking back with you the peaceful and serene feelings.

16. Feel your body in contact with the floor. Remain resting in the Corpse Pose for several minutes, noticing the quality of your breath.

17. Recall your special place, the object you picked up, and its message to you.

18. Gently roll over onto one side, hugging your knees up toward your chest.

19. Transition slowly by gradually returning your body to a comfortable seated position with your eyes closed.

20. Move into the rest of your day slowly and with loving reverence for yourself. Draw upon this sacred place whenever you wish.

My body and mind had been screaming for peace. Through yoga, I found where it had been all along—inside of me.

—LAURA MAZZACCO,
YOGA STUDENT

Yoga has enabled me to experience a calmer state of being, where pressures and responsibilities shrink down to a much more manageable size.

—TERRY HOPKINS,
YOGA STUDENT

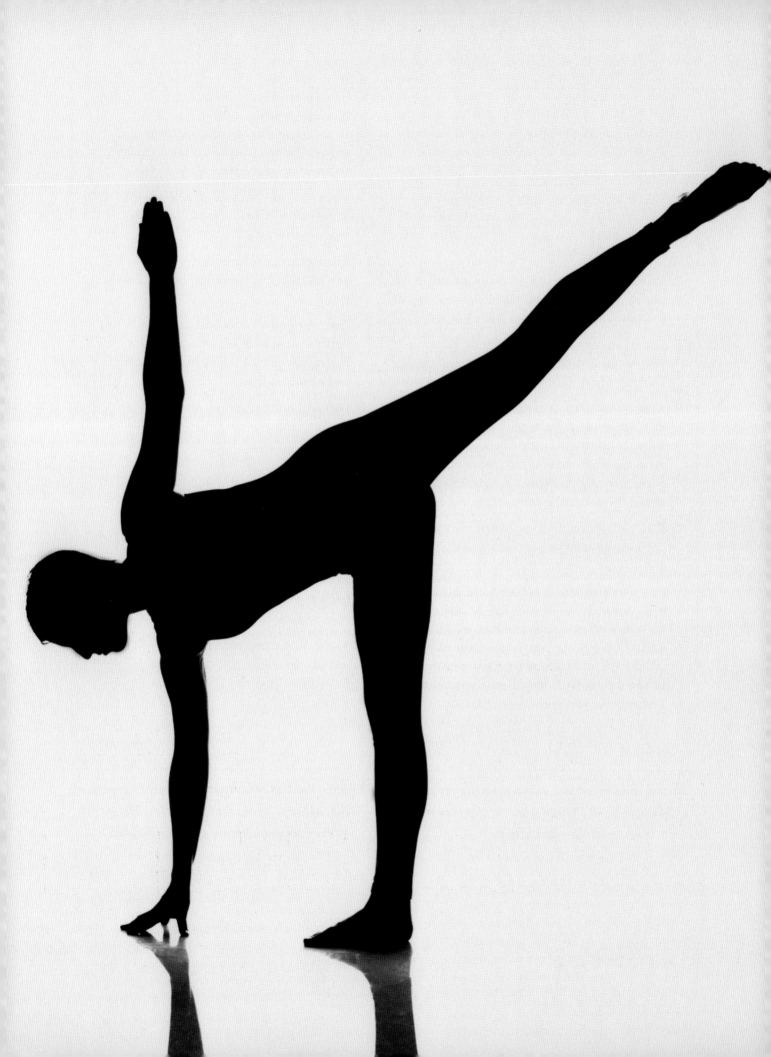

STRENGTH

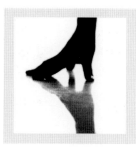

id you ever notice that when you walk on grass, the blades spring back up again? Grass is mowed, raked, and trampled, yet it consistently comes back healthy and green, like a strong warrior who survives battle after battle. This requires resilience and Strength.

Developing the Spiritual Muscle of Strength helps you feel the incredible power of your physical body coupled with the ability to return to your inner core, even after many tramplings. Throughout life, people will be unkind, plans will fall through, things won't always go your way. These are the times when you need to contact the depth of your Strength. Just as physical Strength enables you to carry heavy loads, inner Strength helps you to hold up under burdens that may seem insupportable.

Strength is the balance of will and surrender. If you exert yourself relentlessly, you will eventually burn out. Imagine a body builder who pushes herself to lift weights without allowing for rest and rejuvenation. Along with large triceps and powerful quadriceps, she would soon develop fatigue, injury, and illness.

Many spiritual traditions honor this idea of rest as a way to renew Strength. The assumption is that if God took a break, so should we. The Sabbath, a day set aside for rest and worship, is observed by nearly all religions: on Friday by Muslims, on Saturday by Jews and Seventh Day Adventists, and on Sunday by Christians.

Throughout history, many peoples have been persecuted. There has rarely been a time that Jews have not had to muster up their Strength to face discrimination, destructive enemies, and harsh treatment. Jews maintain the unshakable ability to keep their beliefs going no matter what. Observant Jews draw their Strength from God's law expressed in the Torah, from which they read several chapters a day. By the end of each year, they have read the entire Torah aloud. As Rabbi Harold Kushner says in *To Life! A Celebration of Jewish Being and Thinking:*

> *We don't ask God to change the world to make it easier for us. We ask Him only to assure us that He will be with us as we try to do something hard. . . . If worship is the effort to connect with God, Judaism affirms that we don't have to do all the work alone. God is prepared to meet us halfway. By immersing ourselves in Torah, we transport ourselves to the presence of God.*

Our inner warrior is not a sumo wrestler or a soldier in constant battle, trying to overpower others. Rather, it is a quiet presence whose assistance is always available. The spirit of the inner warrior requires a commitment to integrity, to live passionately, and to trust yourself on a deep level—especially when you feel sensitive.

There is tremendous power in vulnerability. In fact, the word *vulnerability* is related to *vulnerary,* which means "used for healing wounds." The willingness to share your deepest emotions can be a healthy salve, but many people falsely think they are strong only if they never show their feelings. They create an armor of protection against emotions, but this is not true Strength. While armor can be useful at certain times, constant guarding is based on fear, not Strength.

You won't crumble if you cry in public, get angry at a loved one, or feel your own pain. You may believe that if you allow yourself to cry, you will never be able to stop. You *will* stop. And then you will come back like the blade of grass, even more resilient and closer to who you really are.

During this yoga sequence, call upon your perseverance and willful hardiness. Enlist your conscious desire to be in the postures. At the same time, relax into the inherent Strength of each pose. Let go even as you maintain the integrity of the pose. You will tone not only your physical posture and physical muscles, you will also build your stamina to hold any posture (or experience) in life.

Postures for Strength Hara Punches, Warrior II, Inclined Plane, and Up- and Down-Facing Dog all invite you to tap into your power and higher levels of endurance. This sequence is an invitation to sustain your Strength on many levels.

Breathing Lesson for Strength Abdominal Contractions are strengthening and energizing. They help tone the abdominal muscles and connect you to an inner well of resources.

Relaxation for Strength Progressive Relaxation assists you in developing a keen sense of the difference between Strength and tension. This popular technique will also strengthen the immune system.

HARA PUNCHES AND HARA PULLS

Body Benefits:

➤ Rids body of carbon dioxide and stale air from base of lungs

➤ Starts your Strength practice with clean, fresh air

➤ Invigorates and warms body

Let's begin:

1. Come into Proper Standing Alignment but with the legs slightly farther apart than hip distance.

2. Flex the knees slightly to lower your center of gravity and bend the elbows at your sides.

3. With your arms at shoulder height, make strong fists with your knuckles facing out. Take a deep breath in through your nose.

4. Exhale forcefully through your mouth with a "Ha!" as you punch the right fist in front of you. Inhale holding the fist out.

5. Exhale forcefully again with a "Ha!" as you punch the left fist forward, at the same time drawing your right arm back toward your body.

6. Repeat these alternating punches fifteen times, picking up speed as you go along. Be sure to maintain your alignment and try to move only the arms.

7. Now inhale, bringing the arms overhead with fingers open as if to grab Strength from above.

8. As you exhale with a "Ha!", make fists and draw the forearms down in front of you. The elbows should point toward the floor.

9. Repeat steps 7 and 8 fifteen times.

10. When you are done, raise your fists up in the air overhead, holding in the breath.

11. Relax the hands by opening the fists as you exhale slowly and lower the arms down.

12. Close your eyes. Feel your inner Strength.

When to avoid this posture Do not practice Hara Punches if you are pregnant or have high blood pressure, heart disease, or nervous disorders. Stop if you feel dizzy or light-headed.

Yoga Tip *Hara* is the Sanskrit word for the area of the body (around the abdomen) from which life energy emanates. Focus on drawing power from this area as you imagine you are throwing away tensions with each punch. Apply your robust presence to push stress away from your physical and mental being. As you pull your hands to your belly, visualize that you are drawing into your body Strength and energy from the abundance of the universe.

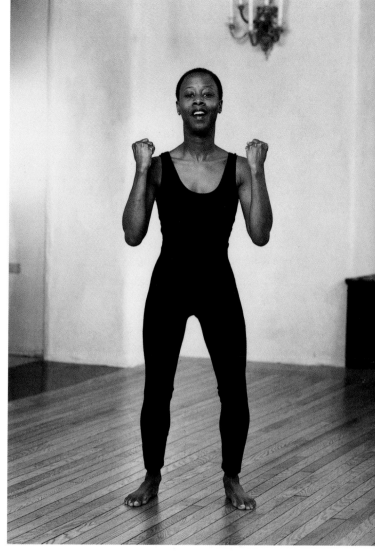

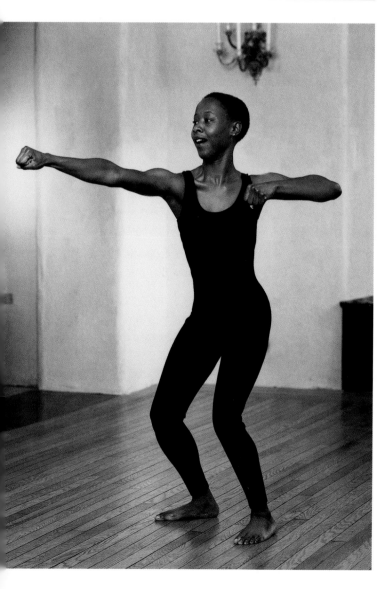

Rather than some kind of dogged pushing through, strong determination involves connecting with joy, relaxing, and trusting. It's determination to use every challenge you meet as an opportunity to open your heart and soften, determination not to withdraw. One simple way to develop this strength is to develop a strong-hearted spiritual appetite.

—PEMA CHÖDRÖN

WARRIOR II

Body Benefits:

➤ Strengthens legs, hip joints, arms, shoulders, and neck

➤ Stimulates circulatory and respiratory systems

➤ Stretches and firms inner thigh muscles

➤ Improves digestion

➤ Helps align spine

➤ Heats and invigorates body

The yogi never neglects or mortifies the body or the mind, but cherishes both. To him the body is not an impediment to his spiritual liberation nor is it the cause of its fall, but is an instrument of attainment. He seeks a body strong as a thunderbolt, healthy and free from suffering so as to dedicate it in the service of the Lord for which it is intended. As pointed out in the Mundakopanisad, the Self cannot be attained by one without strength, nor through heedlessness, nor without an aim. Just as an unbaked earthen pot dissolves in water the body soon decays. So bake it hard in the fire of yogic discipline in order to strengthen and purify it.

— B. K. S. IYENGAR

Let's begin:

1. Begin in Proper Standing Alignment.

2. Inhale, and as you exhale, step the right foot to the right about three feet (about a leg's length apart).

3. Turn the right foot so that the toes point to the right.

4. Turn the left toes to the right just slightly, keeping the hips facing forward.

5. Raise your arms out to your sides at shoulder height, and stretch the hands away from your body.

6. Keep the left leg straight as you bend the right knee and lunge to the right. Be sure to keep your right knee in line with your right ankle.

7. Gaze over your right fingertips and breathe deeply into your belly for several breaths.

8. Imagine that you are a mighty warrior.

9. To switch sides, straighten the right leg and turn your left foot toward the left with the right toes facing in slightly toward the left. Keep the hips facing forward.

10. If you are fatigued, let your hands down in between sides. When you are ready, raise them back up and repeat steps 6–8 on the opposite side.

11. When you are complete, straighten both legs and step the left leg in to meet the right.

12. If you feel steady, you may close your eyes. Slowly lower your arms down to your sides with awareness. Take a deep breath and exhale with a sigh.

When to avoid this posture Hold for only short periods of time if you are pregnant, have high blood pressure, heart disease, or nervous disorders.

Yoga Tip Try to be in this pose with effortless effort. Even though it is a challenging posture, find ways to relax the parts of the body that are not necessary to tense (check your facial muscles and respiratory muscles first). Use your will and call upon the parts of you that *want* to hold Warrior II. Explore various subtleties that enable you to maintain this inherently strengthening posture without struggling.

I myself have no power. It's the people behind me who have the power. Real power comes only from the Creator. It's in His hands. But if you're asking about strength, not power, then I can say that the greatest strength is gentleness.

—LEON SHENANDOAH, SIX NATIONS
IROQUOIS CONFEDERACY

Yoga has shown me that while there may always be a struggle, great or small, it doesn't need to become overwhelming or an end-all. It is just a challenge to be faced and worked through.

—DIANE YANOSH, YOGA STUDENT

121

INCLINED PLANE

Body Benefits:

➤ Strengthens arm muscles, shoulders, and wrists

➤ Stretches and strengthens legs

➤ Activates nervous system

➤ Stimulates thyroid functioning

➤ Opens and lengthens front of body

➤ Strengthens lungs

➤ Heats and energizes entire body

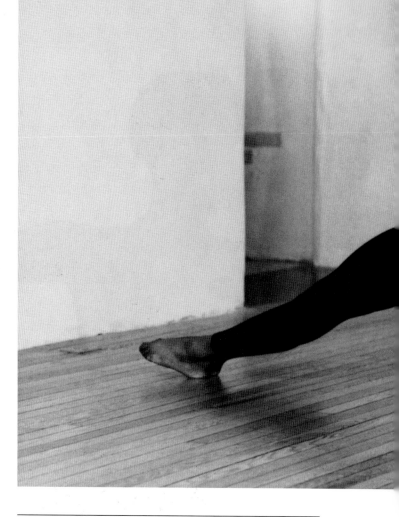

Let's begin:

1. Come into a comfortable seated position with your legs stretched out in front of you on the ground. The toes are flexed toward the face.

2. Keep your spine straight as you rest your hands a comfortable distance behind you with your fingertips pointing at the back wall.

3. With straight arms, press down into your hands and the heels of your feet as you lift the pelvis and the whole front of your body up towards the ceiling. Point the toes away from your body. Look up toward the ceiling.

4. Press the hips as high up as you can, open the chest and keep the buttocks squeezed.

5. If your neck is strong, gently tilt the head back, looking behind you.

6. Breathe into the entire front half of the body. Feel the Strength of your arms and your breath supporting you. Take five to eight breaths.

7. To release, lift the head slowly back up to face forward. Slowly lower the buttocks back down to the ground.

8. Relax the hands in your lap and take several deep breaths with eyes closed as you feel the powerful effects of this posture.

Rock of Ages, let our song
Praise thy saving power
Thou, amidst the raging foe
Wast our sheltering tower
Furious they assailed us
But thine arm availed us
And thy word broke their sword
When our own strength failed us.

—ROCK OF AGES, HANUKKAH SONG

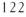

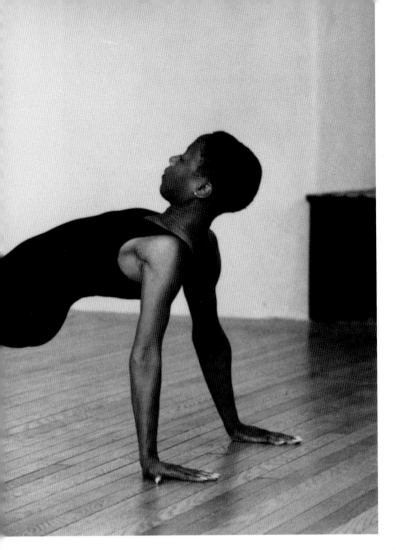

Yoga Tip Be aware of your feelings in the Inclined Plane. Sometimes a certain posture will trigger emotions. Our bodies are storehouses of memory. Some are locked deep inside, while others await you at the door of a posture. You may burst out crying or laughing, suddenly feel angry or filled with love. Don't clog up your emotional arteries by resisting these states. Try to ride them out like waves. They will pass through you and you'll feel stronger, freer, and healthier.

The path of glory is rough and many gloomy hours obscure it. May the Great Spirit shed light on yours.

—BLACK HAWK

UP-FACING DOG

Body Benefits:

➤ Activates abdominal organs, kidneys, and adrenals

➤ Opens, expands, and strengthens lungs

➤ Increases flexibility of spine

➤ Strengthens wrists, arms, shoulders, and back

➤ Relieves menstrual discomforts

When to avoid this posture Do not practice the Up-Facing Dog if you are pregnant or have had recent or chronic shoulder injury or inflammation.

Yoga Tip Physical-Strength training and inner-Strength training are connected. Christiane Northrup, M.D., author of *Women's Bodies, Women's Wisdom* and former president of the American Holistic Medical Association, encourages people to develop bone Strength with weight-bearing exercise. In her *Health Wisdom for Women* newsletter, she explains that women who exercise regularly live about six years longer than couch potatoes—and actually have small but significant gains in bone. In this chapter, you are lifting and supporting some of your body weight. Instead of fearing osteoporosis as the inexorable price of a long life, you can help prevent bone thinning by putting your muscles to work—make no bones about it!

Let's begin:

1. Start in the Table position with your fingers spread apart.

2. Press your pelvis forward so that your legs are straight and resting on the floor.

3. Keep your hands directly under your shoulders and allow your belly to come down toward the ground. Keep your pelvis tucked.

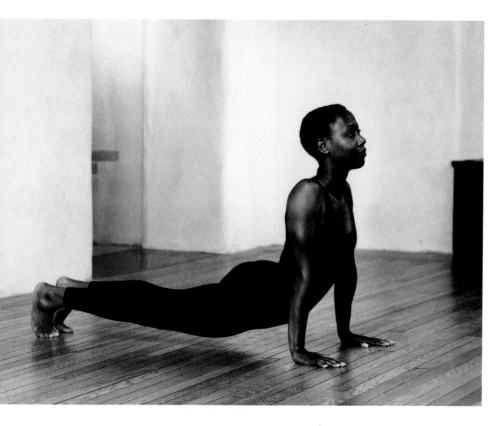

4. You can allow the tops of the feet to remain on the ground, or tuck the toes under and lift up your whole body.

5. Breathe down into the belly.

6. Keep your shoulders broad and your gaze either directly forward or up toward the ceiling.

7. To release, lower the legs back to the ground, then press the hips back into the Table position on all fours.

8. You may wish to counterstretch the spine with the Child Pose.

DOWN-FACING DOG

Body Benefits:

➤ Stretches, lengthens, and strengthens spinal column

➤ Detoxifies entire system when held

➤ Stimulates lymphatic and circulatory system

➤ Opens shoulders and releases tension

➤ Brings fresh blood and oxygen to face

➤ Stimulates proper functioning of pituitary and hypothalamus glands

➤ Improves mental functions, such as memory and concentration

➤ Lengthens and stretches muscles, ligaments, and nerves in backs of legs

When to avoid this posture If you have eye conditions such as detached retina, weak eye capillaries, glaucoma, conjunctivitis, or any infection or inflammation of the eyes or ears, do not practice the Down-Facing Dog.

Yoga Tip If your body came with an owner's manual, it would probably say, "Do the Down-Facing Dog every day to maintain a strong, healthy body." The Down-Facing Dog strengthens several major muscle and joint groups at once: abdominals, hips, thighs, arms, shoulders, and back, as well as your breathing apparatus. And because it increases circulation of blood and lymph, it's also good for the heart muscle. This posture will help you transform your will-o'-the-wisps into acts of willpower.

Let's begin:

1. Start in Table position on all fours with your fingers spread apart on the ground.

2. Curl your toes under and press your hips and sitting bones up into the air, straightening your legs.

3. As you inhale, lengthen your spine.

4. Your head is between your arms, and you are looking behind you through your legs.

5. Try to hold for at least eight to ten breaths so that your muscles lengthen. Focus on pressing the backs of the legs toward the back wall each time you exhale. Engage a subtle form of the back position found in the Cobra.

6. Stretch down the length of your arms while keeping your weight primarily on the legs.

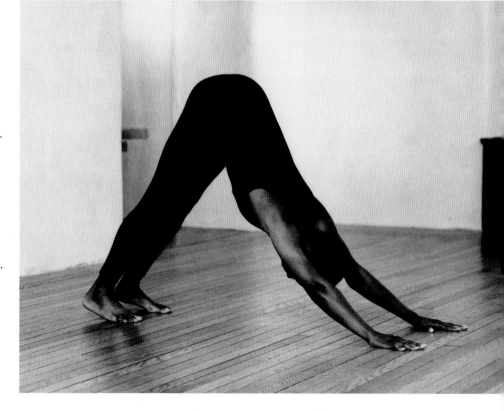

7. Your heels reach toward the floor.

8. To release, lower the knees back down onto the floor returning to the Table position.

Body Benefits:

➤ Tones and firms abdominal muscles and diaphragm

➤ Relieves constipation

➤ Strengthens digestive tract

➤ Strengthens organs and glands that support abdominal wall

➤ Stimulates adrenals, kidneys, and liver

➤ Brings increased elasticity to lungs

➤ Tones heart

ABDOMINAL CONTRACTIONS

Let's begin:

1. Start in Proper Standing Alignment with legs slightly farther than hip width apart.

2. As you inhale, raise your arms overhead.

3. Exhale forcefully through your mouth so that all the air is expelled from the lungs. Sweep the arms and torso forward, lowering your hands to your thighs with your knees bent slightly.

4. With your mouth closed and your *breath held out*, suck your belly and abdominal organs in and

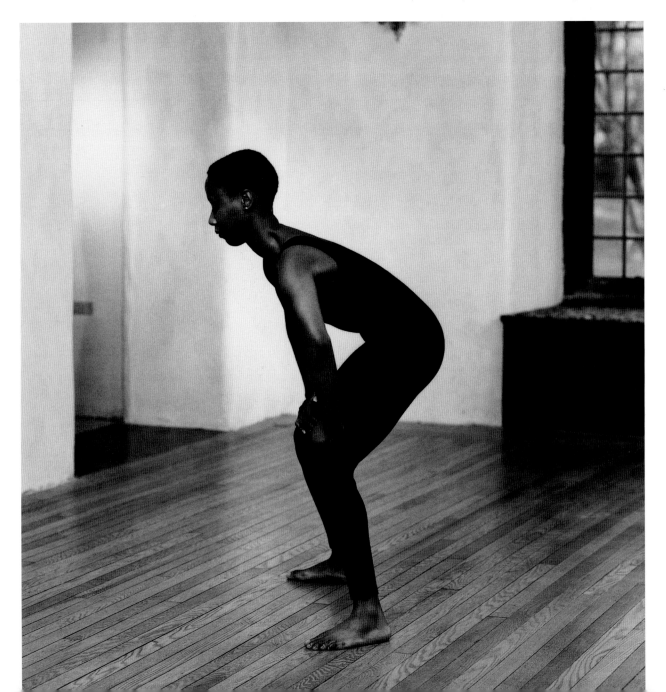

When to avoid this breathing technique Do not practice Abdominal Contractions if you are menstruating or pregnant, have high blood pressure or a history of heart disease or stroke. This technique may loosen an intrauterine birth control device (IUD).

Breathing Tip This challenging breathing exercise takes practice. It involves one of many yogic "locks." Imagine that you have a well of energy in your belly that you are locking in. Once safely sealed in, the pumping action stirs it up so that you can channel it in meaningful, useful ways. Because it is locked in, this energy will not be able to dissipate and leave you feeling tired.

Variation Practice in a comfortable sitting position or on all fours in the Table position.

up toward your spine. You are forming an abdominal cavity.

5. Continue to hold your out breath as you pump your belly back out to the normal position and then quickly snap it back in several times. Start with five pumps and work up to twenty.

6. When you can no longer hold the out breath, inhale to an upright standing position.

7. Allow your breathing to return to normal before you repeat this sequence five more times. You can use the Ocean Breath or the Breath of Fire to facilitate this.

CREATE YOUR OWN POSTURE FOR STRENGTH

Let's begin:

1. Practice the formal postures before creating your own.

2. Begin in a comfortable standing position with your eyes either opened or closed. In your mind's eye, visualize yourself as a warrior.

3. Recall what it felt like to survive past difficulties with success and stamina.

4. See yourself conquering internal battles and enduring current hardships.

5. Begin now to move in ways that represent your inner warrior. How would you move, given an unlimited amount of Strength and power?

6. Move as slowly or as quickly as feels comfortable. With every movement, sense the body's resilience.

7. When you find a position that mirrors your ideal inner warrior, hold it and breathe into your belly. Feel the stamina of this posture in every cell of your body—your legs, your arms, your abdomen.

8. Imagine that you could drink this Strength into your entire being.

9. Make a note of the posture and name it. Compose an affirmation that reflects your inner Strength. Add this to your Strength sessions or create new ones each time.

I visualized myself as so strong that I lifted my queen-size bed with one hand, held it up in the air, and vacuumed under it with the other.

—KATHY MCCOMB-WYKA, YOGA STUDENT

Yoga is a retreat from the storms of life. It re-energizes me and readies me to continue—not as though I were going into battle once again, but as a capable person moving through life.

—RANDI GALANOWSKY, YOGA STUDENT

YOGA STORY FOR STRENGTH: JONJI PROVENZANO

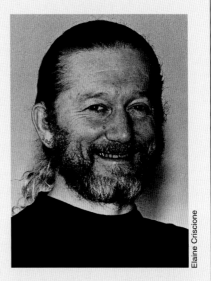

Elaine Criscione

It's challenging enough to practice yoga when you feel healthy and all of your body parts are fully functioning. But what about when you don't feel well—or worse? What if, like Jonji Provenzano, you broke your back?

I decided to open and operate a yoga studio, but I didn't believe that I could support myself without my seemingly secure job as a carpenter/foreman. So I took on some small carpentry jobs. While working on a roofing job, the scaffolding collapsed. I felt my back snap and all of the air blew out of my body.

From inside my head, I heard the word *breathe*. All of my breath training came back, and I took charge of my breath. I used it to cut through the rising tide of panic within me. There I was all alone out in the country, realizing that I had probably broken my back. I knew not to move much, but I spent a few anxious moments seeing if I could wiggle my toes. Then I surrendered into that moment of my life. I let go into this breath, then the next, and the next.

I spent six hours in very intense pain strapped to a hospital board. I was told not to budge. After eighteen hours of holding that posture, I decided to begin the process of regaining Strength in my body. I knew if I didn't start, I might never move again.

It took me an hour to grab a towel that was six inches away. When I finally got it, I twisted it up and made it into a yoga tie that I used to slowly stretch. The nurse yelled at me.

Desperate, I listened to my yoga audio tapes and practiced daily, without moving a *physical* muscle. I simply imagined my body in the postures. I wore a weird metal brace for the next six months.

I continued to develop inner and outer Strength through yoga by honoring my limitations—but still challenging myself. After a year, the daily pain subsided. Two years later, I was pain free, except an occasional reminder to keep me humble and aware of how precious life is.

We can all endure disaster and tragedy, and triumph over them—if we have to. We may not think we can, but we have surprisingly strong inner resources that will see us through if we will only make use of them. We are stronger than we think.

—DALE CARNEGIE

PROGRESSIVE RELAXATION

Relaxation Tip By exaggerating the tension in your body, you will become keenly aware of what it feels like to live in a tight, contracted body. When you totally relax and notice the distinct difference, you'll never want to go back!

Let's begin:

1. Come into the Corpse Pose.

2. Take five deep breaths until you feel relaxed and centered.

3. You will be contracting and tensing parts of the body on an inhalation, then relaxing them on an audible exhalation (a sigh) in a progressive sequence from your feet up to your head.

4. Become aware of your feet. Inhale and tense the feet only, lifting them off the ground slightly.

5. Exhale with a sigh and release the tension and the weight of the feet.

6. Notice the difference.

7. Move your awareness up to the calves and thighs. Lifting them off the ground, tighten them as you inhale and hold the breath.

8. Exhale as you sigh and relax the calves and thighs to the ground.

9. Notice the difference.

10. Shift your awareness into your pelvic area. Squeeze the buttocks, suck the tummy in, and tighten the pelvis as you inhale.

11. Hold, squeeze a little bit more, and then relax. Release your breath audibly along with the tummy, buttocks, and pelvis.

12. Notice the difference.

13. Bring your attention to the lower, middle, and upper back. See if you can isolate these parts as you inhale and contract them.

14. Exhale and release the back completely. Let your back melt into the ground as you notice the difference.

15. Move your consciousness into your chest area. Inhale and contract the chest and hold until you need to exhale.

16. As you exhale, let the chest relax, noticing the difference.

17. Shift your attention to the neck and shoulders. Inhale and contract, squeezing the shoulders up around the neck.

18. Exhale with a sigh, then let the shoulders drop and the neck release. Notice the difference.

19. Focus now on your arms and hands. Clench your arms, lifting them slightly off the ground. Make fists as you inhale.

20. Exhale through the mouth and relax the arms down to the ground, uncurling the fingers.

21. Let your arms be heavy on the floor. Notice the difference.

22. Shift your attention to your facial muscles. Inhale and contract your face as if it were a raisin. Squeeze your eyes tight, furrow your brow, scrunch up your cheeks and your mouth.

23. Exhale and totally relax and let your facial muscles go. Notice the difference.

24. Now inhale, squeezing and contracting your whole body, from the feet to the crown of your head. Lift the arms, legs, and head slightly off the floor. Exaggerate the holding. Tense the entire body.

25. When you are ready, release and exhale with a giant "Aaah." Let the body go. Allow your breath to come in and out of your relaxed and revitalized body. Become an astute observer of the difference between held tension and relaxed Strength.

26. Rest, simply breathing for several minutes.

27. As you feel ready, roll your body over onto one side, hugging your knees up toward the chest. If any tensions come back, simply breathe into them.

28. Gently bring your body back up into a comfortable seated position, returning to your day with a deep sense of inner Strength.

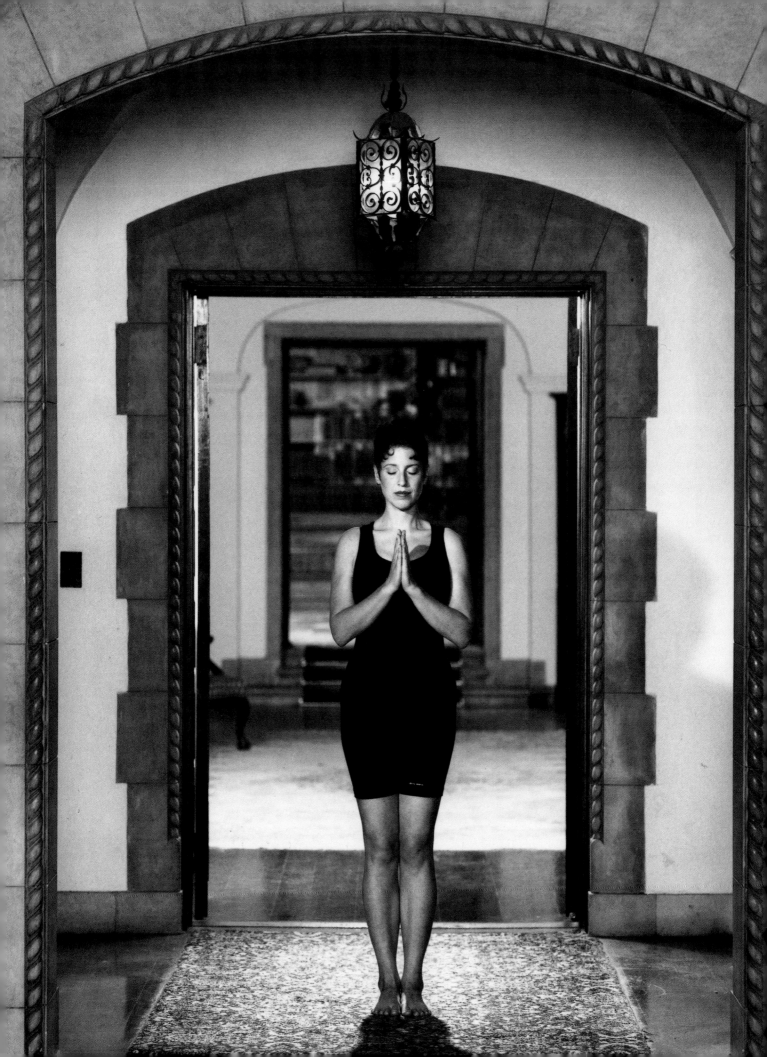

COMPASSION

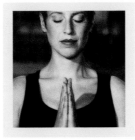

"We are the world!" go the lyrics to the popular song. Whatever happens to others—or the world—happens to us, and vice-versa.

As we embrace the world's pain as our own, we exercise the Spiritual Muscle of Compassion. Imagine that you are the Earth. Is your head at war with your body, creating internal strife? Do you have a deep and chronic ache in the Middle East section? Are there areas of your inner atmosphere that are polluted or clogged up?

All beings suffer, hurt, need, and feel lonely. Simply being alive makes us candidates for Compassion. To develop the Spiritual Muscle of Compassion means to feel empathy for other beings, both those we know and perfect strangers, those we love and those with whom we have differences, as well as ourselves. It is a way of understanding, a means of saying, "I know where you're coming from," a way to walk in another's shoes.

Through most mass media, we are confronted daily with images of war, crime, hunger, and other tragedies. Much of the time we numb ourselves to them. You may wonder, "I don't even know those people. They live three thousand miles from me. How could I possibly make a difference?"

The Talmud teaches, "If you save one soul, it is as if you saved the whole world." You must believe that you are not separate from others. Those hungry children could be your children. Their losses could be yours.

We can begin a local practice of Compassion with those directly around us. By understanding their problems, being an empathic listener, offering support when they are in need, you are helping everyone. Moreover, your behavior will be a role model for others to inspire their instincts for Compassion.

While you are being compassionate toward others, don't forget yourself. To develop self-Compassion, listen to your body carefully and make efforts to respond to it. On days when you are sick or tired, lovingly offer yourself the same care you would any other human being. Be gentle and take the bird's-eye view of the situation. Observe yourself as you would your best friend: "She's so tired. She's pushing to the point of becoming ill. She needs to rest and take care of herself."

Tonglen is the Buddhist practice of giving and receiving Compassion. There are many stages of Tonglen practice. One of the preliminary exercises is

We must widen the circle of our love till it embraces the whole village;
the village in its turn must take into its fold the district, the district the province,
and so on till the scope of our love becomes coterminous with the world.

—MAHATMA GANDHI

called Self-Tonglen, where you imagine yourself divided into two parts, A and B. A is the loving and unconditional friend within, while B is the hurt child or the part of you that feels upset and wronged. Inhaling, you imagine that A generously allows B into her heart. Exhaling, B can open her heart as the pain is lessened with this powerful acceptance.

If we could all practice self-Compassion, we would be filled with the Compassion necessary to flow out into the rest of the world. Compassion is limitless, boundless, and transformative. To actively practice Compassion requires courage. Most spiritual teachers are the embodiment of Compassion and practitioners of their own form of Tonglen. Jesus, Gandhi, Mother Teresa, the Buddha, the Dalai Lama, Thich Nhat Hahn, and endless others represent Compassion in action.

In Sogyal Rinpoche's clarification of *The Tibetan Book of Living and Dying*, it says, "Compassion is not true compassion unless it is active. Avolokiteshvara, the Buddha of Compassion, is often represented in Tibetan iconography as having a thousand eyes that see the pain in all corners of the universe, and a thousand arms to reach out to all corners of the universe to extend his help."

Practice loving-kindness through your thoughts, actions, words, and intentions. Allow yourself to look through eyes of Compassion rather than indifference. Let your hands offer a caring touch. Know that your body and mind are the doors to uncovering the depth of Compassion that lies within all of us. As we discover the healing capacity of self-Compassion through yoga, we awaken our inherent desire to surround another being's darkness with light.

Yoga teaches us how to embrace the world with Compassion. By putting ourselves into many different yoga positions, we are better able to understand the variety of human experiences. By breathing into uncomfortable sensations and feeling tightness and tensions, we can learn about our fears, limits, and attachments. They have a lot to teach us. We must have mercy for ourselves and for all sentient beings. We are all in this together.

Postures for Compassion Child Pose I and II, Legs-Up-the-Wall Corpse Pose, and Knee Hugs are symbolic postures of self-love. While the Fish opens our hearts to the world around us, Gentle Head to Knee helps us embrace our own hearts. Throughout this or any other chapter, feel free to use pillows or cushions under any part of the body that calls for extra attention.

Breathing Lesson for Compassion Compassion Breath allows the energy of your heart to radiate out to the rest of your being.

Meditation for Compassion The Temple of Compassion is a way to bring loving-kindness into every aspect of your life.

The quality of mercy is not strained;
It droppeth as the gentle rain from heaven
Upon the place beneath. It is twice blest;
It blesseth him that gives, and him that takes.

—WILLIAM SHAKESPEARE, FROM *THE MERCHANT OF VENICE*

YOGA STORY FOR COMPASSION: JAGANATH CARRERA

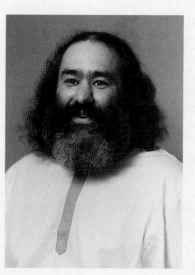

Reverend Jaganath Carrera bases his life on many of the messages of his spiritual teacher, Swami Satchidananda. "Never miss an opportunity to serve" is his guiding principle. He created additional opportunities by helping to organize a new concept, a yoga ministry. The first ordination was in 1980. He has served at Rutgers University within the campus ministry and is now the president of the Integral Yoga Ministry Board.

I wanted to make a deeper commitment to the spiritual teachings and be able to serve people in more ways—but I wasn't called to monastic life. Being a minister of yoga has helped me take the teachings of yoga into the world. One of best ways I gauge my growth spiritually is by how much Compassion I feel.

It's easier to feel the Compassion that dwells within me when I do meditation, deep breathing, and postures that open up my chest and heart. Yoga's job is to help free the areas that are blocked so that I can be in touch with my deeper self. The Compassion is already there; yoga helps us contact it.

Yoga also teaches the tools to put Compassion into action. The real challenge arises when someone treats you with anger or accusation. One time a woman applied for the ministry and I had to tell her that she should wait another year and then reapply. She accused me of being biased against her. I realized her feelings were a result of her disappointment and pain. Years later, when we met again, I treated her with love and kindness, which initially shocked her and then softened *her* heart. Opening my heart through yoga helped open the doors of our friendship again. It was quite amazing!

As I get to know myself through yoga, I realize we are all more alike than different. Yoga develops clarity and strength of mind. If I have a weak, fearful mind, I won't be compassionate. I must be strong enough to leave myself and meet the other person. I also try to be compassionate with myself. Compassion is not the martyr syndrome. The true power of Compassion begins to appear when you expand your human family to the point that you feel there are no more strangers in the world.

I feel as though I have been a tightly closed bud and now I am beginning to blossom . . . unfolding petal by petal, reaching for the warmth and nourishment of spirit.

—AILEEN MURPHY, YOGA STUDENT

CHILD POSES I AND II

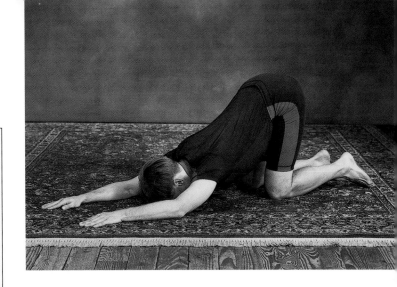

Body Benefits:

➤ Counterstretches back-bending poses

➤ Normalizes circulation and respiration

➤ Relaxes and flexes spinal ligaments and muscles

➤ Aids reproductive and digestive functioning

➤ Improves circulation to brain, pelvic area

Let's begin:

CHILD POSE I

1. Begin by kneeling, sitting on your heels. (If this is difficult, place a cushion on your calves.)

2. Folding at the hips, bring your chest toward your knees. Rest your forehead on the ground or as close to the ground as is comfortable.

3. Stretch your arms out in front of you on the floor. Or rest them alongside your body, palms up.

4. You may want to rock the hips from side to side to release tension in the lower back.

5. Remain in the Child Pose for several full, deep breaths. Bring your awareness to your heart, which is lovingly surrounded by your body.

6. To release, press into your palms and lift the torso back up to a kneeling position.

CHILD POSE II

1. Begin in the Table position with your hands directly under your shoulders and your knees beneath your hips.

2. Slide your hands out in front of you along the ground. Walk them as far out as you can.

3. Lower your torso and rest the forearms and forehead on the floor.

4. Take several deep breaths and enter a state of quietude.

5. To release, either slide your hips back to Child Pose I or walk your hands back up into the Table position.

6. When you have completed the Child Pose series, come into a comfortable seated position and place your hands over your heart to reconnect to its healing energy.

Yoga Tip These two poses are positions of rest, so make them as comfortable as possible. You may need to have a cushion or a rolled-up blanket under your hips or forehead for Child Pose I so that you can relax your pelvic weight into the cushioning. If your abdomen is large, spread your knees to accommodate the extra room needed.

Let Child Pose II be a prostrate ritual of reverence. Let the energy from your heart flow down through your hands, extending Compassion out to all brothers and sisters in the world family. In both postures, invite your mind to descend into your heart.

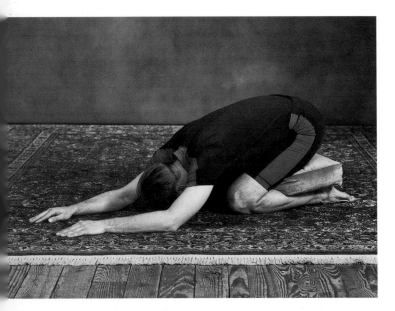

LEGS-UP-THE-WALL CORPSE POSE

Body Benefits:

➤ Reduces tension and swelling in legs

➤ Allows blood and lymph fluid into abdomen

➤ Stimulates circulatory system

➤ Lowers blood pressure in medicated mild hypertension

➤ Brings relief to tired, over- or underworked legs

When to avoid this posture Do not practice Legs-Up the Wall Corpse Pose after the third month of pregnancy. Avoid it if you are at risk for miscarriage, are menstruating, or have a hiatal hernia or sciatica.

Yoga Tip As you do this posture, visualize the energy from your legs flowing down into your heart—the center of Compassion. Imagine that you are collecting a sacred pond of love that cascades down the waterfall of your legs. Enter a devotional state and allow your open arms to symbolize your openness to divine love.

Let's begin:

1. Sit on your buttocks with your legs out in front of you. Your right hip and right shoulder are against the wall.

2. Lie down and swing your legs up, at the same time pivoting your body ninety degrees. Scoot your buttocks up as close to the wall as you can, so that your legs rest straight up.

3. Allow your hands to rest by your sides, palms up. Let all of the blood drain out of the legs, giving them a minivacation.

4. Imagine that your back is melting or sinking into the ground.

5. Breathe slow, steady, deep breaths as you lie in this inverted Corpse Pose for as long as you like.

6. When you are ready to release, bend the knees in toward your chest with your feet against the wall. Let your legs flop down to the left. Gently press your torso back up into a seated position.

7. Place your hands over your heart as you feel the deep integration of this posture.

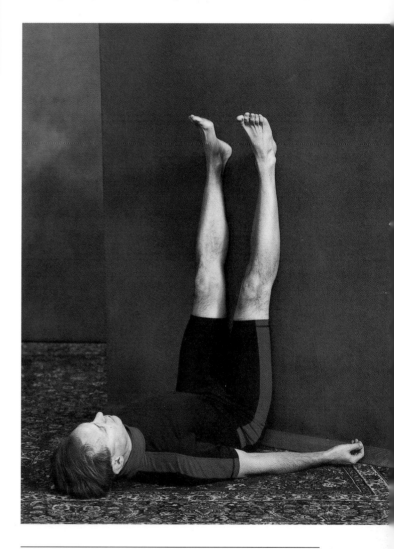

It is only with the heart that one can see rightly; what is essential is invisible to the eye.

—ANTOINE DE SAINT-EXUPÉRY

KNEE HUGS

Body Benefits:

➤ Helps cure and prevent flatulence

➤ Stimulates peristalsis

➤ Induces state of relaxation

➤ Improves flexibility in hips

➤ Relaxes spine

When to avoid this posture If you are pregnant, do not practice Knee Hugs.

Yoga Tip Studies show that touch stimulates the immune system, alleviates depression, energizes, decreases stress, and increases the amount of hemoglobin (which carries life-giving oxygen to the organs) in the blood. Many researchers have demonstrated the therapeutic use of touch. Dr. Tiffany Field of the Touch Research Institute studied premature infants. Babies who were massaged fifteen minutes a day gained almost 50 percent more weight than those who did not receive this growth-stimulating touch. Healing touch is also available through the language of hugging. According to such hugging advocates as Dr. Leo Buscaglia, no one can have too many hugs a day. Hugging yourself counts!

Let's begin:

1. Come into the Corpse Pose.

2. Grasp your right leg midshin and hug your knee into your chest.

3. Lift the head and bring the forehead as close to the knee as possible. Breathe comfortably.

4. Be conscious of keeping the lower back pressed into the ground. If you feel any discomfort at all in the lower back, bend the left knee and place the left foot on the floor with the right foot resting on the left thigh.

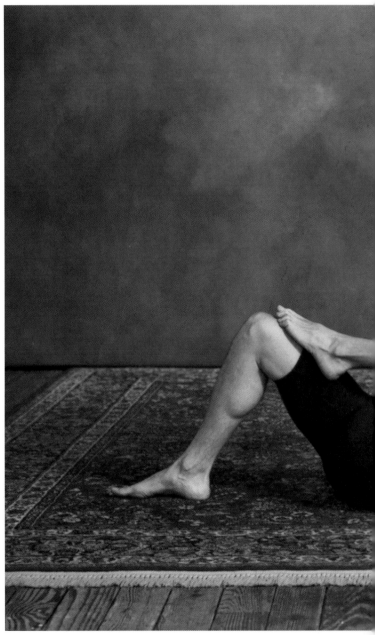

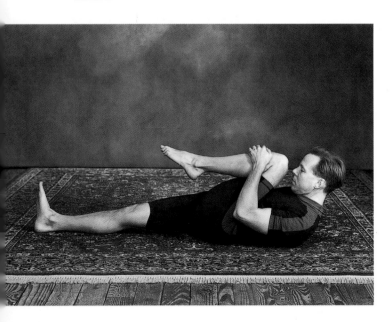

5. Hold for five to ten breaths and focus all of your attention on this self-nurturing hug.

6. Release the head and right knee. Take a few moments to rest in the Corpse Pose. Note the differences between the right and left sides of the body.

7. Repeat steps 2–6 with the left knee.

8. After you have completed both sides, rest in the Corpse Pose for several breaths with your hands over your heart.

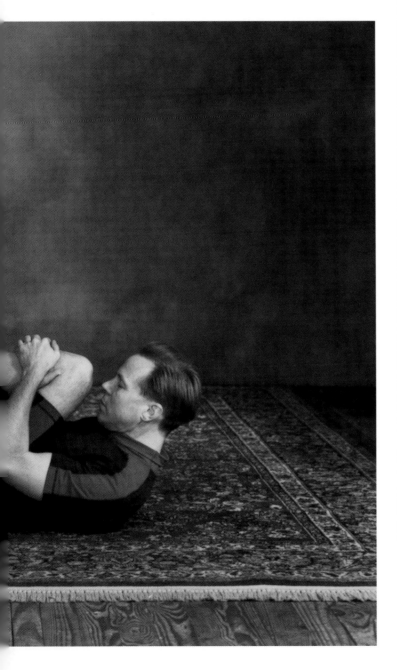

CREATE YOUR OWN POSTURE FOR COMPASSION

Let's begin:

1. Practice the formal postures before creating your own.

2. Begin in a comfortable seated position with your eyes closed. Wrap your arms around your shoulders in a big hug. Slowly release, taking several deep breaths.

3. Consider a situation, person, or event that you feel Compassion toward. Sense that you are welcoming that person or situation into your heart. Feel yourself embracing it as you would a crying, hurt child. Acknowledge your longing to alleviate suffering.

4. With your eyes closed, allow yourself to move in ways that embody your deep understanding and love for this being or event. Allow your movements to tell a story of your deep concern. Let your body's message be a prayer in motion.

5. When you find a position or movement that you want to hold, stop moving or repeat the movement several times. Stay here for several breaths.

6. Make a note of the posture you have created and give it a name. Create a positive affirmation of your heartfelt Compassion that you can repeat when you are in this posture. You may wish to draw a picture or write about it. Add this to your regular practice. Allow this posture to help you discover deep understanding on a visceral level.

FISH

Body Benefits:

➤ Expands chest area, increasing lung capacity

➤ Helps respiratory ailments including asthma

➤ Stimulates thyroid functioning

➤ Flexes and strengthens neck and entire spine

➤ Improves functioning of reproductive organs, liver, spleen, and pancreas

➤ Soothes nervous system

➤ Normalizes adrenal functioning

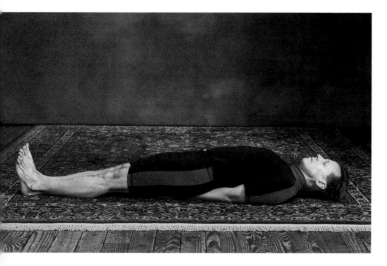

Sometimes teaching must be strong. Compassion is not only gentleness. A sharp blow of the . . . stick of awakening, placed just right, is also an act of compassion.

—TAISEN DESHIMARU,

FROM *THE RING OF THE WAY*

Let's begin:

1. Start in the Corpse Pose. Roll your body side to side as you walk your straight arms underneath the body and try to hide the elbows. Your palms and forearms are turned down. If this is too challenging, simply rest the arms beside your body with palms down. In both instances, draw your toes back toward your face.

2. Press down into the forearms and lift the torso up off the ground. Gently place the crown of your head on the ground, looking behind you. Keep your weight on the forearms. Breathe into the open chest and heart. You are now balancing on the crown of the head, the forearms, buttocks, legs, and heels.

3. If your neck is strong, release the support of the forearms by walking your arms out from under your buttocks and back. Bring the hands into prayer position over the chest. Use the lift in the chest and the sitting bones to take the weight off your head.

4. Hold for five to ten breaths as you allow Compassion to wash over you.

5. To release, return your forearms back to a supportive position close to your body. You may wish to grab hold of your hips or the outsides of your upper thighs. Release the head by pressing into the forearms and rolling the spine back onto the ground—lower back first, then the upper back, and finally the back of the head.

6. Return to the Corpse Pose.

7. Become aware of the quality of your breath. Relax here for several moments with your hands over your heart.

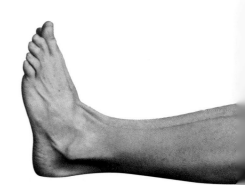

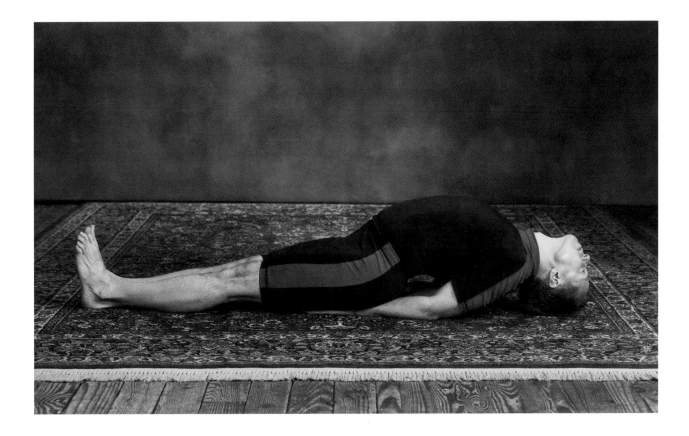

When to avoid this posture Do not practice the Fish if you have had recent or chronic neck injury or inflammation.

Yoga Tip Many traditions refer to seven *chakras*, or major energy centers within the body. *Chakra* is a Hindu word that means "wheel of light." This posture opens up the heart chakra. Imagine a beautiful green (the color of the heart chakra) light bathing your heart and surrounding your entire body. You may sing the sacred sound of this chakra, which is "Yam." As you repeat this sound, feel the vibration in the heart area.

For many folks, this posture is challenging at first. Be gentle as you open up to the strength and vulnerability of your being. Take the Fish in stages. At first, you may be able to go only as far as step 1 or 2. With practice, you will be surprised at how much more comfortable you become with the Fish.

GENTLE HEAD TO KNEE

Body Benefits:

➤ Stimulates digestion and relieves constipation

➤ Stretches and flexes spine and hips

➤ Energizes and decongests nervous system and abdominal organs

➤ Improves circulation throughout reproductive system, upper body, and legs

➤ Stimulates proper functioning of pancreas, liver, gall bladder, kidneys, spleen, intestines, gonads, and bladder

➤ Promotes hemorrhoid relief

When to avoid this posture If you have recent or chronic hip or leg injury or inflammation, do not practice Gentle Head to Knee. If you are pregnant, come into the pose only as far as is comfortable without putting pressure on the belly.

Yoga Tip This posture is usually done with a straight, outstretched leg. Because our model Stephen injured his knee, we adopted this pose into a less strenuous version of the classic Head to Knee. Show Compassion toward yourself during this or any posture. In Gentle Head to Knee, you may not only bend the knee, but also place cushions under the knees and/or hips. As you glide your torso forward, sense your heart extending out as an offering of love to the world.

Let's begin:

1. Assume a seated position with your right leg straight out in front and slightly to the right. Flex the toes of the right foot back toward your face, and maintain a lengthened spine.

2. Bend the left knee, tucking the left foot in toward the inner right thigh and groin.

3. Lift the arms overhead with palms facing, fingertips together.

4. Shift the torso to face the right leg.

5. Hinge at the hips and maintain a flat back as you reach forward over the right leg. Hold at various points, breathing deeply.

6. When you can no longer come forward with a flat back, bend the right knee as much as required in order to bring the head down close to it. Round the spine, bring the chin to the chest, and rest the hands as far down the right leg (or toes, if you can) as possible.

7. Hold onto the right leg and breathe into this soothing posture until you reach your toleration point.

8. To release, leave the arms down and let them slide up your legs. Slowly roll up the spine, stacking one vertebra on top of the other. Or if your back is strong, reach the hands and arms forward and come back up with a straight spine.

9. Repeat steps 1–8 on the opposite side.

10. Once you have completed both sides, sit upright with legs stretched out in front of you. Place your hands over your heart to connect with how you are feeling at this moment.

Do not hurt your neighbor, for it is not him you wrong but yourself.

—THE SHAWNEE

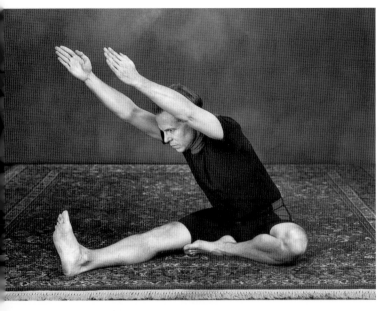

*The stress of feeling that I had to perform
to the same level as others in the class
was erased by the simple instruction,
"Listen to your body."*
—J O Y   V A N D E R   V L I E T ,
Y O G A   S T U D E N T

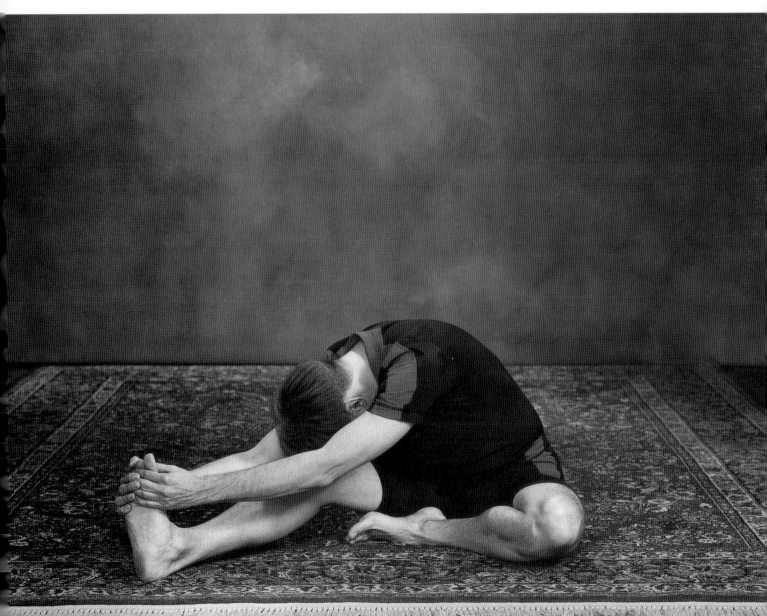

Be still my heart, wherever I am, I am at home with you.

—ZULU CHANT

COMPASSION BREATH

Yoga Tip Many temples in China, Korea, and Japan are dedicated to Kuan Shih Yin, the symbol of divine Compassion. Kuan Shih Yin means She-Who-Hearkens-to-the-Cries-of-the-World. Tara is a Buddhist goddess of Compassion who is said to have been born of the Buddha's tears of Compassion. As you practice this breath, think of yourself as the embodiment of Compassion.

Let's begin:

1. Come into Proper Sitting Alignment with your eyes closed.

2. Inhale deeply. As you exhale, sigh it out, "Aah." Take several of these long and soothing breaths.

3. One atop the other, place your hands over your heart. Feel the drumbeat of your heart. Become absorbed in the rhythm of its pulse.

4. As you connect to the energy of your heart, imagine it spreading across your entire body—through your arms and legs, swirling around your torso and into your head.

5. Imagine the loving energy of your heart filling up every cell of your being. Each time you inhale, gather loving heart energy into your heart and palms. With every exhalation, the energy spreads to each and every cell.

6. Inhaling, collect this healing gift in your heart. As you exhale, allow it to radiate out and surround your body with its protective power. Feel it encompass your entire being, encircling your head, face, and neck all the way down to your sitting bones.

7. On the exhalation, let this energy flood the parts of your body that might feel uncomfortable, achy, tight, or uncomfortable. Send your Compassion-infused breath to all parts of you.

8. From a deep inner smile, let a slight smile light your face.

9. When you feel complete, return your hands back in your lap. Notice the connection between your hands and loving heart even when they are not touching.

10. Inhale and then exhale with a sigh, "Aah." Repeat three more times.

11. Notice how you feel at this moment. Allow your eyes to open very slowly.

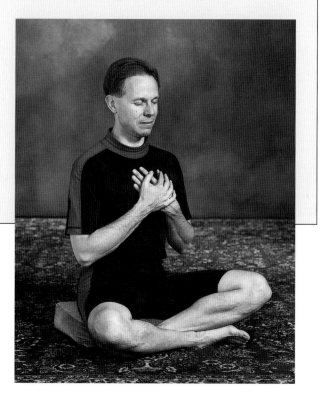

I feel like I'm breathing more of the world in.

—MARY JEAN IPPOLITO, YOGA STU-

DENT

TEMPLE OF COMPASSION

Yoga Tip Before you begin this loving experience, take a moment to sit quietly. Using your thumb, rub the center of the opposite palm with gentle circles. Repeat on the other hand. This is an accupressure point that directly relates to the heart. It's also a special treat when done with someone else. I used to sit with my grandfather and massage his hands while he told me stories. Hand massage is a healing and soothing experience alone or when practiced on others.

1. Come into the Corpse Pose. Take several full and deep breaths.

2. Imagine that you have a temple inside your heart. This is the Temple of Compassion and houses healing love. Kindness, mercy, light, and wisdom live here.

3. In your mind's eye, picture what this temple looks like: its size, shape, what it's made of.

4. There are steps leading up to the Temple of Compassion. See yourself at the foot of the steps and then proceed up to the main door. When you are ready, walk through the door and rejoice in the splendor of this magnificent temple.

5. Spend several minutes here. Feel yourself being embraced by the deep understanding that lives in this hallowed space.

6. Now invite in loved ones, friends, family, and pets. See them ascending the stairs to the temple and passing through the door. Welcome them and allow them to absorb the energy of conscious Compassion. Greet or embrace them in any way you wish.

7. Feel free to invite anyone who is no longer living, your ancestors, a place that you love, or anything or anyone else that has significance in your life.

8. If your temple feels big enough and generous enough today, invite those people or situations with whom you have difficulty. Watch them come up the stairs and through the doors of loving-kindness.

9. Now allow all sentient beings into your temple. Know that there is plenty of room to fit the entire universe. See the world's animals, plants, and flowers gracing your beautiful temple. Allow sick, hungry, lonely, and frightened beings to find a safe, loving, open sanctuary. Welcome newborn infants, children, adults, and older people of all shapes, colors, and nationalities.

10. Sense the openness and receptivity of your heart. Know that to the extent your heart is available to yourself and others, to that degree you will attract Compassion back to yourself.

11. Remain in your temple as long as you wish. Sanctify this place in your heart and bring it back into your daily life experience.

12. When you are ready to return from this meditation, gently deepen your breath. Feel your body in contact with the ground beneath you.

13. Slowly roll over onto one side hugging your knees to your chest. Gradually bring yourself back up into a comfortable seated position. Be still and silent until you want to open your eyes.

14. You may wish to journal about your experience. Express any feelings of ease or difficulty. Let your journaling be a ceremonial act of respect that acknowledges your whole experience.

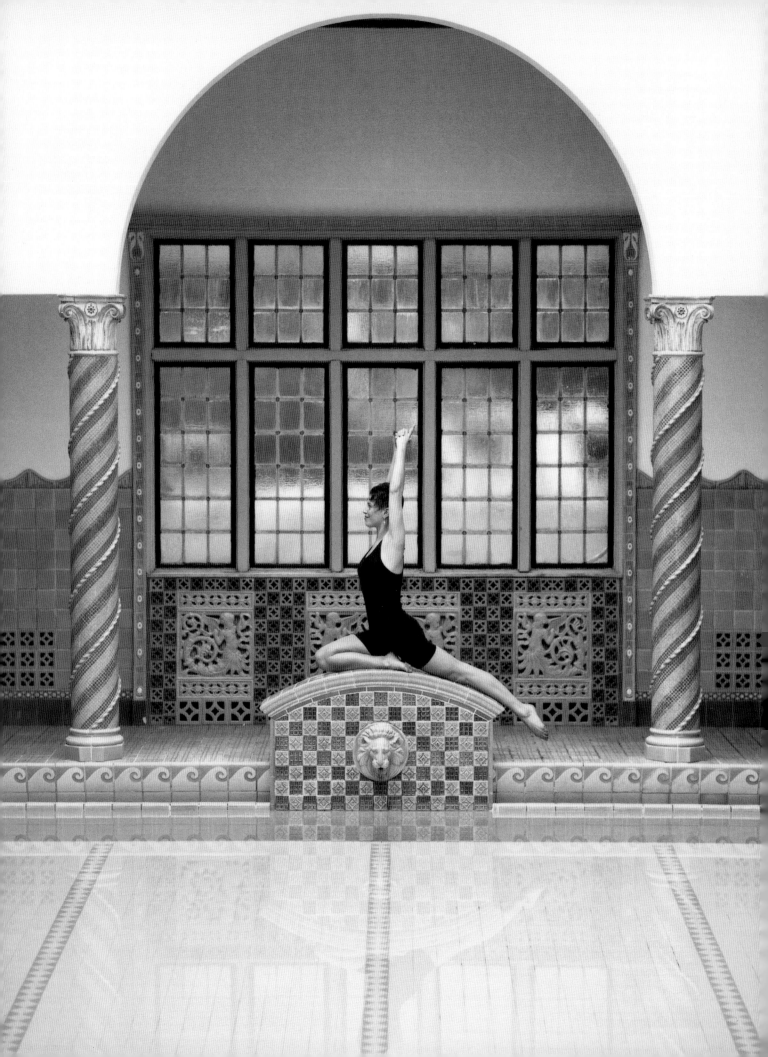

ENERGY

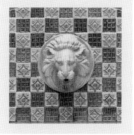

One of the biggest misconceptions about our source of Energy is that it's "out there somewhere." The truth is that Energy is within us, ready and waiting for us to access its supercolossal potential. Our life Energy is an innate intelligence that masterminds everything from healing wounds to maintaining our breath while we sleep. This Energy within us is part of the ocean of universal Energy that governs all life. We can tap into it through our individual currents.

Our culture doesn't have a word for this life force Energy. The Chinese refer to it as *chi* or *qi,* while *prana* is its equivalent in India. The Japanese call it *ki,* meaning the "seat of the soul." Some employers in Japan analyze a prospective employee's ki to see if it's strong enough to handle the job. In ancient Greece, life Energy was called *pneuma,* which means "breath."

The ways that we breathe, think, eat, work, and move all contribute to the quality of Energy that manifests in our lives. Breath is an essential link to our vitality. By consciously directing it, we can calm anxiety, awaken our innate vibrancy, and induce states of heightened awareness. Breath control is as powerful and potent as artificial substances.

Within each of our bodies is a fully stocked apothecary. In fact, the words *body* and *apothecary* are derived from the same root. Drugs only mimic what the body can do naturally. We don't need to take drugs to feel the enthusiasm and invigorating

enjoyment of Energy. Simply by getting excited about life or entertaining positive, compelling visions, our bodies automatically produce hormones that boost our vitality and have a positive effect on the immune system. The field of knowledge known as psychoneuroimmunology studies how negative thought and anxious worry drain Energy and how positive, life-enhancing thoughts boost our resistance to disease.

As ideas are food for thought, literal food is Energy for life. The fuel we put into our bodies is what feeds the spirit. The word *vegetable* comes from the Latin, meaning "to animate or enliven." *Spirit* has the same definition. When we are deficient in Energy, it can mean that we lack some form of nutrition.

The very act of eating is a spiritual experience. Many people pray over their food in gratitude and as a way to imbue it with healing Energy. In order to sustain our creative Energy, we need to take

Dig within. There lies the well-spring of good: ever dig, and it will ever flow.

—MARCUS AURELIUS

responsibility for the inner atmosphere we create through eating. In the natural foods cookbook *Kripalu Kitchen,* Levitt, Smith, and Warren state, "As prana is a form of energy at work in our bodies, we need to replenish its activities; thus we take in food which contributes its own prana or life-giving energy to us. This is then transformed in our bodies from gross physical matter into more subtle energies, producing movement, heat, thought, and activity."

We have all enjoyed times when we've felt truly nourished and energized by a meal. Similarly, we have all endured moments when our choices have dragged us down and depleted our Energy. That which sustains our animating essence comes not only from what we feed it, but also from what we *don't* feed it.

Sometimes, *not* eating for short periods can be enlivening. Overtaxing the body without giving it a break, like never changing the oil in your car, creates a buildup of dirt and residue. When we purify the diet or briefly fast, we give our systems a rest, a chance to heal from abusive habits. Jews on Yom Kippur, Muslims at Ramadan, and many other cultures observe holy days by fasting. During those times when we choose to be empty, we can be filled with spirit.

Filling up every moment of your day and working yourself to the point of exhaustion drains your Energy. Tired or sick animals instinctively rest, whereas humans tend to run themselves ragged trying to do just one more thing. Wasting our vital resources in this way is similar to leaving your car headlights on and running down the battery. Avoiding burnout keeps your body's battery charged. Learn as much as you can about your own Energy cycles by listening and responding to your body's messages.

Play with yoga postures at the edge—not so far that you strain yourself nor so effortlessly that you are unchallenged. This healthy edge is different for everyone. It also varies within an individual from day to day, depending on a multitude of factors from emotional fatigue to how much sleep you've had.

Tensions are often stored-up Energy. Encountering tensions is a normal part of the process of yoga. Yoga permits us to recycle this power so that it is freed up for productive and useful purposes. We maximize our potential, transforming daily life into opportunities for experiencing more aliveness.

Postures for Energy Energy Squats are a great warm-up for the dynamic movements in the Warrior Series. The Pigeon helps you draw up Energy from the Earth. A program for invigorating body, mind, and spirit would not be complete without the Half-Bow and the Bow.

Breathing Lesson for Energy The Breath of Fire is a powerful technique that, once learned, can be used in a pinch. If you are worried about falling asleep at the wheel, pull over and practice this breath. You will be amazed!

Visualization for Energy Body of Energy awakens your enthusiasm and zest for life.

Every feeling is a field of energy. A pleasant feeling is an energy which can nourish.
Irritation is a feeling which can destroy. Under the light of awareness, the energy of irritation
can be transformed into an energy which nourishes.

—THICH NHAT HANH

YOGA STORY FOR ENERGY: ANAMIKA COLEMAN

Anamika Coleman is a ball of Energy. Everything she does with her life, from yoga to teaching Kripalu's DansKinetics™ to Shiatsu massage, is connected to Energy and spirit—which she shares generously with anyone in her radiant presence.

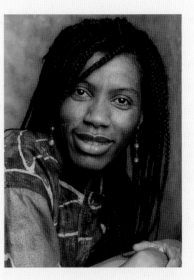

In the late 70s and early 80s, I traveled around Norway as a disc jockey. City to city, catching planes and late nights were a way of life for me. It was a fast-paced, busy, and rather unhealthy atmosphere in the discos. Often exhausted, I took naps in the afternoons. Little things bothered me, and I often made them into big issues. I was reactive and occasionally explosive. I loved playing the wonderful music and considered myself a "conscious disc jockey," but I knew I needed a shift. I had a lot of Energy, but I didn't know how to channel it.

Then I started to study yoga, and it has become my haven. My work purpose shifted and drastic changes began occurring in my body and my emotions. Yoga balances my Energy and transforms it into a calm strength. It helps me maintain a high-Energy life. I now know how to work with my Energy, how it flows, and what stops it from flowing. When I'm in a stressful situation, I breathe and unblock the Energy.

Lately, I do only one or two postures and then I sit and simply breathe. I maintain a straight spine so the Energy can travel freely. Once you take on the commitment of yoga, the payoff is great. Since I've been practicing yoga for fifteen years, I'm really reaping the benefits. It's like having a DNA print of the postures inside of me that I can tap into.

The DansKinetics™ that I teach and helped to develop is a combination of dance, aerobics, and yoga. I call it the Dance of Yoga, as you are moving from the inside out. We use dynamic, energizing music that takes you into a place of deep feeling. I introduced African dance and drumming to the program. The drumbeat, like the heartbeat, reminds us that we all belong to the Earth. It brings us back to our primal existence. We want to be barefoot and move naturally. It awakens the Energy within us and we feel charged.

Yoga is like my breath, and without breath, you can't live. It's what keeps me going. There's a powerful vitality in people who practice yoga and acknowledge their spirits. If we don't feel energized and *really* alive, nothing else in life is worthwhile.

Beseeching the breath of the divine one, His life-giving breath,
His breath of old age, His breath of waters, His breath of seeds,
His breath of riches, His breath of fecundity, His breath of power,
His breath of all good fortune, Asking for his breath
And into my warm body drawing his breath, I add to your breath
That happily you may always live.

—ZUNI CHANT

ENERGY SQUATS

Body Benefits:

➤ Stimulates digestion

➤ Strengthens ankles, calves, and hamstrings

➤ Improves complexion

➤ Aids memory

➤ Increases flexibility in pelvis

➤ Brings fresh oxygen to brain

When to avoid this posture If you are pregnant or have glaucoma or detached retina, uncontrolled high blood pressure, or a history of heart disease or stroke, keep your head above your heart. Do not allow your head to hang down in the Rag Doll, but instead follow the variation described in step 3.

Yoga Tips In many cultures, the Squat is a habitual way to sit. It is the natural position for childbirth. As children, we naturally squatted. Sitting for long periods of time on sofas, in cars, and on desk chairs has shortened our muscles. For some, the squat is extremely difficult. For others, it's simple. Our bodies are all built differently. Delight in the differences! Don't worry about what your squat looks like. Who cares?

I love the Rag Doll. Your body naturally opens and stretches while it simultaneously relaxes. Let go of the muscles in your neck when you do the Rag Doll. Let your head hang down. When you hold tension in your body unnecessarily, you drain Energy. Let yourself just hang, doing nothing, and you will have more Energy for the things in your life that really matter.

Through yoga, I have learned how to find the energy that is hiding within me, waiting to be found.

—HANAN ABBASSI, YOGA STUDENT

Let's begin:

1. Start in a Squat with your knees bent and your buttocks hanging down between your legs. Keep your spine straight. With your arms inside the knees, rest your hands on the floor. Your heels may be flat on the ground or you may be up on your toes. Your feet can be far apart or close together. Your body will decide best how to squat. Take a few full breaths.

2. On an exhalation, press the hips up into the air. You may or may not be able to keep your hands on the floor.

3. Let the upper body hang in the Rag Doll with the legs straight or knees bent slightly (do not lock the knees). Feel your torso spill out of your waist. Let the head hang down so that the top of your head is reaching toward the floor. **Variation:** As you lift your hips up from the Squat, place your hands or elbows on your bent knees with your back flat and parallel to the ground. Keep your head in line with your spine; do not drop your head below your heart.

4. Repeat this movement from Squat to Rag Doll several times. Begin slowly and work up to a faster pace. Inhale into the Squat and exhale with an open mouth "Ha" into the Rag Doll.

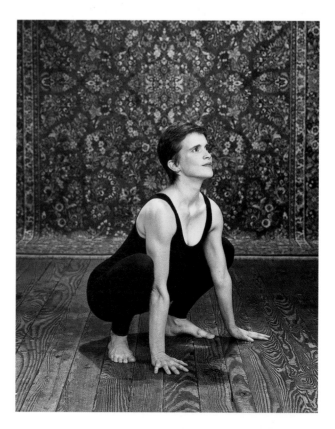

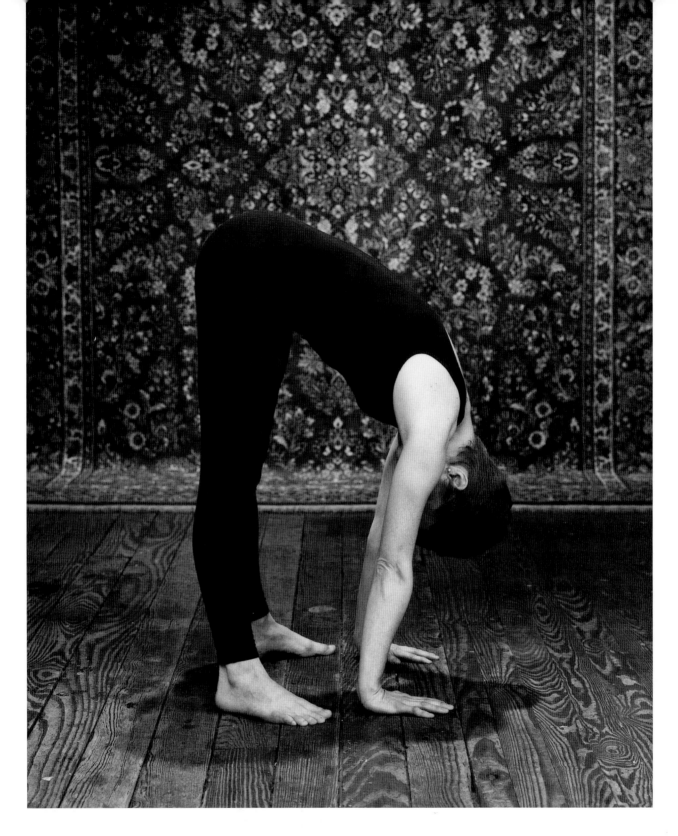

5. To return to standing, bend the knees, tuck the tailbone under, and stack your vertebrae one on top of the other. Keep your chin on your chest until you are fully standing. Finally, lift the chin to come into Proper Standing Alignment. Allow your breath to normalize.

6. Keep your eyes open until you feel steady. If you feel a head rush, take a minute to sit down or touch a wall to help you balance.

7. Close your eyes and experience the newfound Energy awakening in your body.

WARRIOR SERIES

Let's begin:

1. Come into Proper Standing Alignment with your hands on your belly. You will be moving into the various warrior movements on the exhalations and returning to this position on the inhalations.

2. With your hands on your belly, take a deep breath through the nose.

3. Exhale through the mouth with a "Ha" sound. Simultaneously, lunge the *right* leg forward and sink down into the right bent knee. Lift the arms overhead with the palms facing each other into Warrior I. Keep the knee directly over the ankle.

4. Inhale through the nose as you lunge back to the starting position with your hands over your belly.

5. Exhale through the mouth with a "Ha" sound, lunge the *left* leg forward, and sink down into the left bent knee. Be sure to keep the knee directly over the ankle. Simultaneously, lift the arms overhead, palms facing each other, into Warrior I.

6. Inhale through the nose as you lunge back to the starting position with your hands over your belly.

7. Exhale through the mouth with a "Ha" sound as you step the *right* foot a leg's length to the right, bending both knees. Simultaneously, draw your arms up overhead, bending the elbows at shoulder height with the palms facing each other in the Victory Pose.

8. Inhale through the nose as you lunge back to the starting position with your hands over your belly.

9. Exhale through the mouth with a "Ha" as you step the *left* foot a leg's length to the left, bending both knees. Simultaneously, draw your arms up overhead, as you did in step 7.

10. Inhale through the nose as you lunge back to the starting position. Simultaneously, interlace your hands at belly level and draw them up overhead, palms facing out.

11. Exhale, bend the knees, lower your arms in front of you. Return your palms to the belly.

12. Inhale again and draw your interlaced hands overhead a second time, palms facing out.

Body Benefits:

➤ Stimulates circulatory and respiratory systems

➤ Stretches and firms inner thighs

➤ Energizes and decongests nervous system

➤ Improves digestion

➤ Strengthens and reduces stiffness in legs, hips, arms, shoulders, and neck

➤ Helps align spine

➤ Heats and invigorates body

When to avoid this series Do not hold any of the postures for long periods of time if you are pregnant or have uncontrolled high blood pressure, heart disease, or nervous disorders.

Yoga Tip In yogic philosophy, the anatomical location of life Energy is centered just below the navel. Your human battery resides in this area of the lower belly and is the place from which your most powerful passions and emotions arise. As you return your hands to this Energy center each time, imagine that you are drawing vitality from this special place to help you move into the next pose. Interestingly, this is the part of the body where you were first given life (through the umbilical cord). Draw on it at this stage of your journey for life-giving Energy.

13. Finish by exhaling and bending the knees. Lower your interlaced arms, returning your palms to the belly.

14. Straighten your knees and return your hands to your sides in Proper Standing Alignment.

15. Repeat this series and experiment with different paces and holding times.

16. When you have completed one to five rounds of this series, close your eyes and check in. Resist the urge to shake off the Energy. Instead, remain still and allow the Energy to remain in your body.

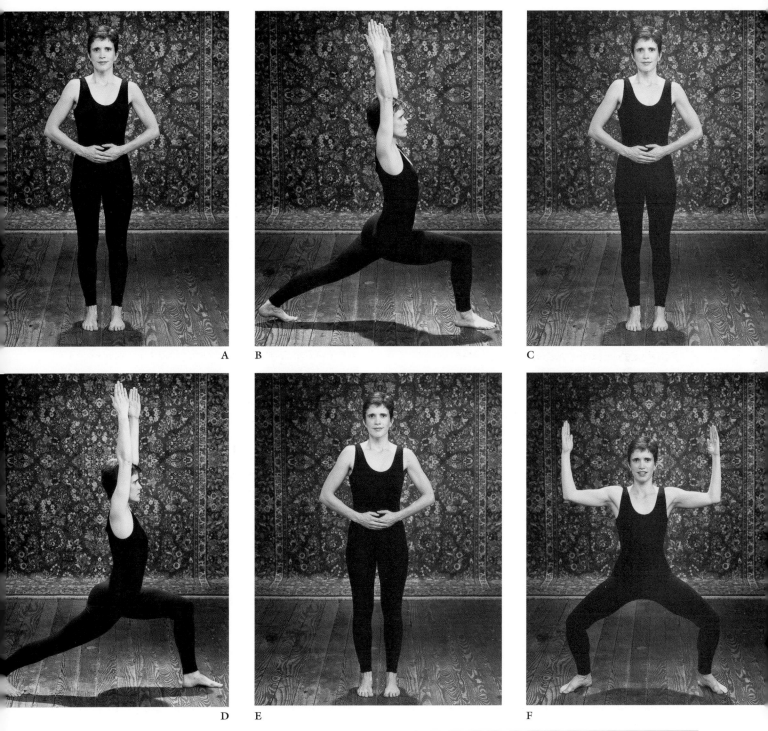

A B C

D E F

I went to an engagement party with my daughter tonight. I've always loved to dance but as I got older, I would get out of breath and sort of gave up dancing—until tonight. I danced every dance, all kinds of dances. My daughter was exhausted and I was still dancing. One woman said to me, "Thank goodness for my aerobics class. It helps to keep up." I said, "Thank goodness for my yoga class." My stamina was unbelievable. I am doing things that I thought were impossible!

—ANNE TYRPAK, YOGA STUDENT

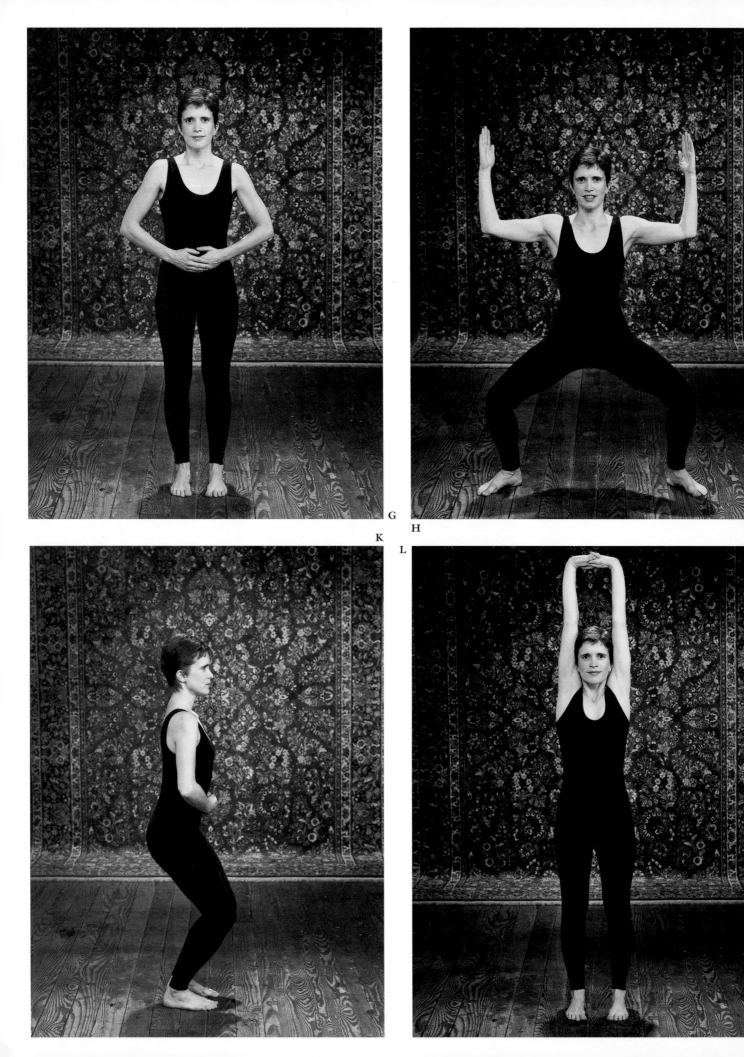

G

H

K

L

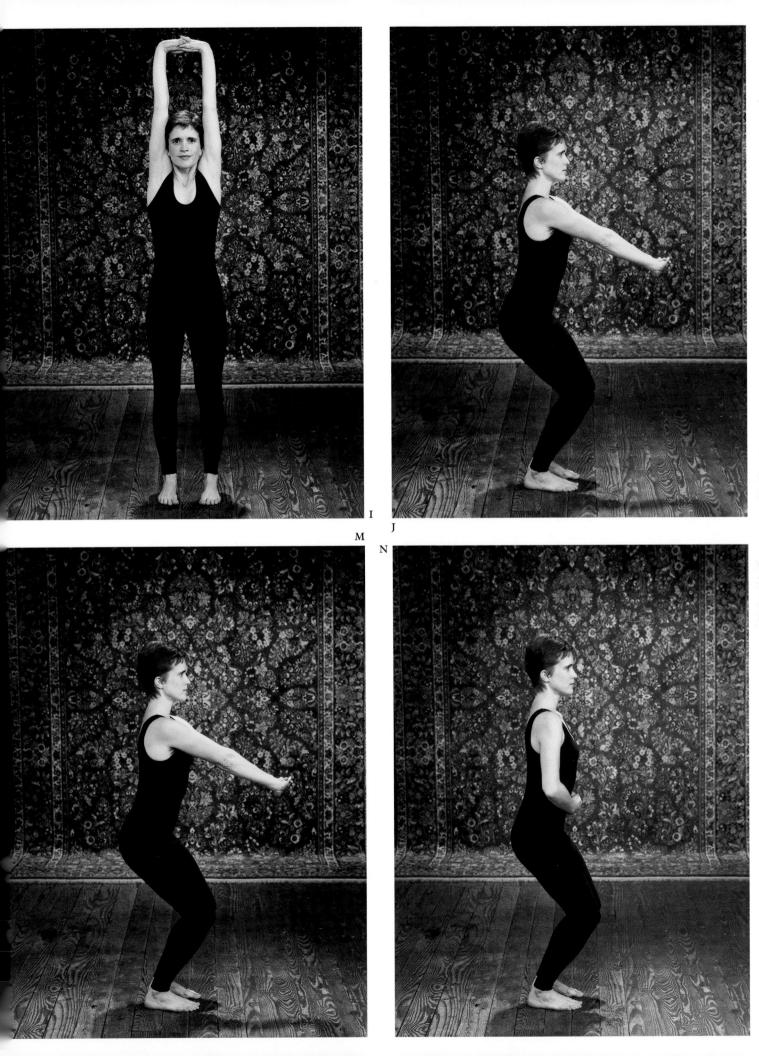

I

J

M

N

PIGEON

Body Benefits:

➤ Provides greater flexibility in hips

➤ Brings oxygen supply to pelvis

➤ Improves respiratory functioning

➤ Tones back muscles and stimulates kidneys with fresh blood

➤ Stimulates endocrine, nervous system

➤ Improves circulation, warms and energizes body

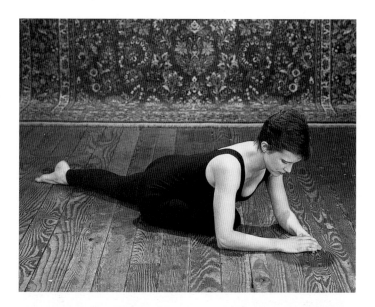

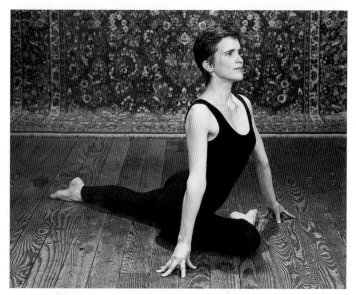

Let's begin:

1. STAGE ONE: Come into the Table position on hands and knees.

2. Extend the left leg straight behind you along the floor with the right shin resting on the floor. With the support of your hands on either side of your bent right knee, lower your torso down over the knee. Keep your head in line with your spine and rest on your elbows with palms together in front of you. (If you are more flexible, you may bring the right foot across to the left side of the body so that you rest on the *outside* of the right lower leg.)

3. Slowly wiggle and shift your hips from side to side using micromovements. Bring your attention to the areas that are tight. If you are able, lower your head to the floor in front of you. Take several deep breaths in this position.

4. Now, rest your fingers alongside the right bent leg and press the torso into an upright seated position, keeping your legs where they are.

5. You can keep the right leg bent and directly under your pelvis. For a deeper stretch, draw the shin and foot farther away from the body.

6. Lengthen up through the crown of your head and breathe deeply into the entire front of the body. Keep the shoulders relaxed and down. Use the abdominal muscles to help you maintain this graceful lift.

7. This is the first stage of the Pigeon. Get comfortable with this stage before moving on to Stage Two.

8. STAGE TWO: Press down into the right bent shin for support. Using the strength of your stomach muscles once again, draw the arms up overhead. The fingers are laced in the steeple position with index fingers pointing up.

9. Breathe deeply, allowing the breath to swell up into the chest. Hold for five to ten breaths.

10. To release, slowly lower the arms back down to your sides supporting your torso.

11. Lift the hips and draw the right bent leg back to meet the left as you return to the Table position.

12. Repeat steps 2–11 on the opposite side. One side

will probably be tighter than the other. Simply notice it without judgment.

13. When you have completed both sides, come back to the Table position. Bring your body down onto your belly in a frontal Corpse position (face down on your belly with the head resting to one side).

14. Check in and notice what happened in the hips and the rest of your body. Do you have more Energy? Do your hips feel freer? Take several moments in the facedown position to stretch the body out in whatever way feels good to you.

Yoga Tip Most adults have tight hips. We carry a lot of trapped Energy in them. The Pigeon helps you to unlock this well of Energy by freeing the hips of tension. Your hips are the biggest joints in your body. Slowly play with micromovements in this posture. The key to getting joints loosened is rotation. Remember: tight places *want* to open, loosen, and relax. Your hips will thank you for it.

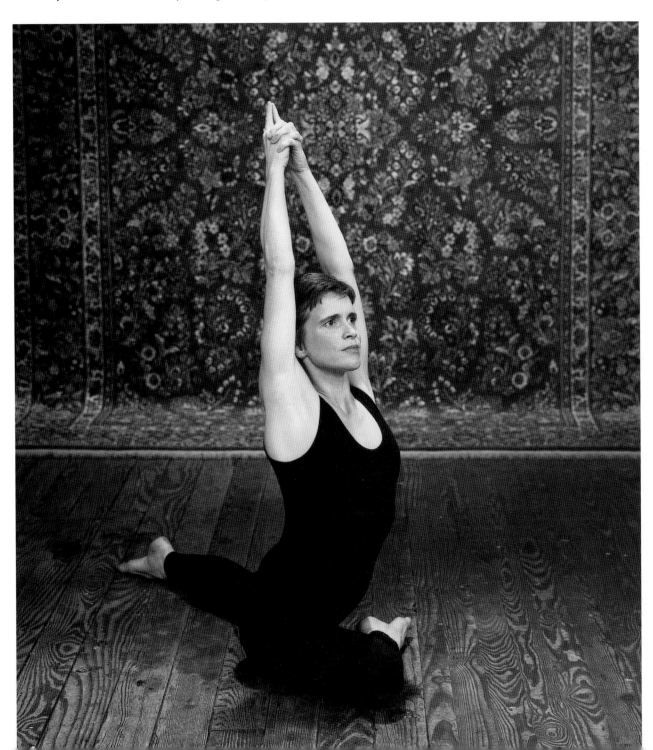

HALF·BOW

Body Benefits:

➤ Energizes entire body

➤ Firms and strengthens buttocks, legs, and abdomen

➤ Heats body and improves circulation

➤ Expands lung capacity and opens chest

➤ Provides kidneys with fresh blood supply

➤ Strengthens back muscles

➤ Stimulates endocrine system

➤ Improves spinal and shoulder flexibility

➤ Aids menstrual disorders

➤ Stimulates and improves digestion

When to avoid this posture Do not practice the Half-Bow during pregnancy, menstruation, if you have had recent abdominal surgery or abdominal inflammation, or have hyperthyroid conditions.

Yoga Tip According to Chinese medicine, all of the meridians, or circuits of Energy in the body, have terminal points in the feet. The Chinese created a map on the bottoms and sides of the feet to show where each part of the body has a corresponding point. Rub the bottoms of both feet and around the ankles without worrying about technique. Foot reflexology is great for the lymphatic system, and it will help heighten and balance your Energy.

Let's begin:

1. Lie down on your belly.

2. Press your upper body off the floor, supporting yourself on your elbows. Shift the right forearm slightly toward the left for better support.

3. Bend the left leg at the knee and point the toe. Reach back with your left arm and grab either the outside or the inside of the foot, depending upon which feels more natural.

4. Keep your focus downward and your pelvis on the ground.

5. Squeeze the buttocks as you kick the left foot up, lifting the left hand. The leg lifts as the arm straightens.

6. Keep the breath moving as you engage in this dynamic pose. Hold for five to ten breaths. See if you can do this *and* smile at the same time. Smiling requires less Energy than frowning!

7. To release, slowly lower the leg, bending the elbow.

8. In slow motion, release the hand from your foot and allow the leg to float back down toward the ground.

9. Lower the torso to the ground and turn your head to one side, relaxing completely.

10. Repeat steps 2–9 on the opposite side.

11. Once you have completed both sides, rest on your belly with your head to one side and relax. Become aware of any shifts in your Energy.

BOW

> **Body Benefits:** See Half-Bow

Let's begin:

1. Lie down on your belly.

2. Keep the buttocks squeezed. Bend both knees. One hand at a time, reach back and clasp either the outside or inside of the ankle. Try to keep your knees approximately hip distance apart. The farther they are, the easier it will be.

3. Take in a deep breath. As you exhale, press down into the pelvic triangle (the two hip bones and the pubic bone) and kick the feet into the hands. The higher you kick, the straighter your arms will be. Point the toes.

4. You can leave your knees on the floor or you can come more fully into the pose by lifting the knees off of the ground as shown.

5. Hold for three to ten breaths. This is a challenging pose and will take time to get accustomed to. Be patient with yourself.

6. To release, with buttocks squeezed, slowly lower your thighs back onto the ground.

7. Gently release your feet and allow your legs to rest on the ground as you lower the torso down.

8. Once you have come back to the original position, turn the head to one side. Close your eyes, release the squeeze in the buttocks, and rest. You may want to windshield-wipe the lower legs from side to side or in and out (in either the American or the European version).

When to avoid this posture same as Half-Bow

Yoga Tip This powerful pose presses down on your belly's Energy center, giving it a satisfying massage. Be sure to keep your breath fluid and full. Savor the release slowly as fresh blood and oxygen rush in to bathe the vital organs. What a gift for the kidneys, which receive a jump start on their job of freeing the body from burdensome waste. In the Orient, the kidneys are considered sacred because they distribute life Energy throughout the body.

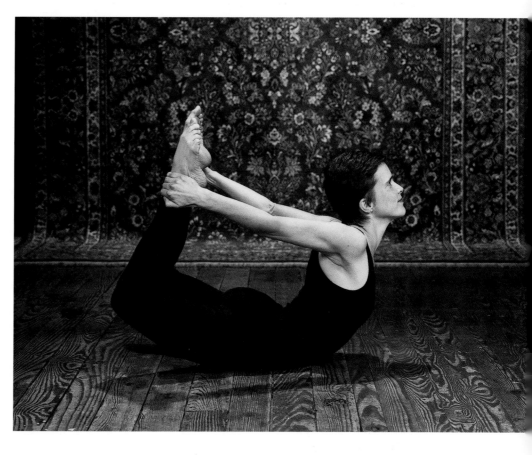

9. To counterbalance the back bending, fold your hips back to your heels into the Child Pose. Allow your breathing to return to normal.

10. Sense the surge of Energy flowing through your body.

CREATE YOUR OWN POSTURE FOR ENERGY

1. Complete the formal postures before creating your own.

2. Come into Proper Standing Alignment. Still your body and mind as you take several full, deep breaths.

3. Place your hands on your belly and close your eyes. Imagine that inside your belly is a ball of Energy. This is your life force.

4. Feel the ball beginning to swirl, roll, and undulate with the Energy of the universe.

5. Sense this Energy within as you slowly roll your hips, bend your knees, and move in whatever way the ball of Energy leads you.

6. Sense the pulse of Energy within you. Connect with the universal, primordial Energy. Do you sense warmth, fullness, or inner calm?

7. Now let your hands, arms, and any other part of your body begin to explore freely.

8. If you find a position that your body wants to hold, stop moving. Stay in this position for several breaths. Open your eyes if you wish. If you sense that the Energy wants to keep moving, allow yourself to continue its dance. Your body will tell you when it's ready to stop.

9. If you found a specific posture to represent your Energy, make a note of it by drawing or writing about it. Give it a name. Create an affirmation that supports your desire for Energy in your life. Repeat this statement while you hold your posture. Add it to your regular practice. If you repeat this experience, you will find that it is different each time.

COLLEGE PRESSURES: YOGA, TAKE ME AWAY!

To be a student requires a wide range of skills, discipline, and concentration. Many students have test-taking anxiety and fear about oral reports and become overwhelmed with how best to prioritize the work that piles up on them. Stress burnout is one of the most common "diseases" on the college or university campus. Just handling the registrar, financial aid, and all the paperwork requires Energy, perseverance, and a sense of humor. The following are some ways to integrate yoga into your student life:

1. Oral presentations are difficult for most everyone. Practice yogic breathing and ingrain Proper Standing Alignment into your visceral memory to help you present your talk with enthusiasm and self-assurance.

2. Before you sit down to study, practice a few rounds of the Sun Prayer to prepare your body and mind. Developing simple but powerful rituals helps to set the tone for a more relaxed and focused academic experience.

3. Instead of trying to keep yourself awake with stimulants, listen to the needs of your body. If it really needs to sleep, studying longer isn't going to help you acquire much more information. Or, try the Breath of Fire to keep yourself alert.

4. Study marathons are not as productive without taking short, energizing breaks every hour or so. Stretch your muscles and stimulate circulation. Hang in the Rag Doll for a minute to send oxygen-rich blood to your head—that's where your brain is! Your memory will also improve with increased oxygen.

5. It's hard to have confidence when you don't do well on an exam or have been up all night to write a last minute term paper. Practicing yoga can help you build self-esteem by developing good posture and alignment, by mastering difficult poses, and by learning how to breathe properly.

6. As your mind expands through learning, don't forget your body. It needs attention too, and will function much better if you give it a stretch. Great ideas and insights often come to me during yoga practice when I'm not even trying.

7. Practice relaxation skills. Another complaint reaching epidemic proportions on college campuses is panic attacks. If things are truly out of control, seek professional help from the counseling center on campus. Continue to support yourself by learning relaxation skills.

8. Share what you learn with the people you love. One of my students dedicated his entire yoga journal to ways that yoga helped him improve his romantic life with his girlfriend. They replaced watching hours of television with time spent breathing together and practicing partner yoga. Their communication improved and they enjoyed a deeper intimate relationship.

9. Sleep disorders haunt many students' lives. Part of this complicated and intricate problem stems from not being able to let go of the myriad thoughts in your active mind. You may find that when you lie down, you can't shut off your brain. Some of my students listen to relaxation tapes to ensure a good night's sleep before they go to bed.

10. If you tend to become anxious or over-whelmed with juggling all of the aspects of college life, take your emotional temperature. Close your eyes for ten seconds, take a few deep breaths, and check in with how you feel. This quick check-in can make a big difference in how you approach the rest of your day.

11. Each time you begin a yoga session, put your book bags aside. With them, leave due dates, responsibilities, research paper ideas, and everything else. Use this time to take a break from your role as a student.

12. When spring break is too far off, practice the Inner Sanctuary Meditation and take a holiday in your imagination. You'll feel relaxed, refreshed, and best of all, you'll get an inexpensive vacation.

13. College life can be lonely, especially if you are on a large campus. Invite a classmate to join you in yoga practice. It can be twice the fun. Or, do what Mike Thiruvillakkat did as a resident assistant at Montclair State University: instead of a Toga Party, have a *Yoga* Party! Mike fostered a yogic atmosphere where the pressures of student life were replaced with lighthearted and meaningful togetherness. "We came together through the yoga postures, and really got into the relax-ation. The party was definitely a success! With healthy food and a noncompetitive attitude, we all went back to studying for finals with an upbeat spiritual tune-up."

14. It's easy to become overly serious when you have more to study and read than seems humanly possible. Smiling is a simple way to release tension. As Vietnamese Buddhist monk Thich Nhat Hanh says in *Present Moment Wonderful Moment*, "A smile can relax hundreds of muscles in your face, and make you master of yourself. That is why the Buddhas and bodhisattvas are always smiling."

15. "Being better able to prioritize and take one thing at a time" is one of the most common benefits I hear from my college students. By practicing Focus in yoga, you will be more equipped to Focus on staying centered in your student life. You'll decide what needs to be done first and what can wait, and you'll maintain your composure during exams.

BREATH OF FIRE

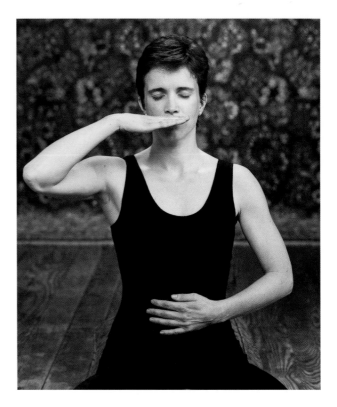

Body Benefits:

➤ Energizes entire system

➤ Cleanses lungs and respiratory system

➤ Purifies sinuses

➤ Activates digestion

➤ Aids constipation and overall elimination

➤ Strengthens abdomen and diaphragm

➤ Clears mind

➤ Aids memory

Let's begin:

1. You may want to blow your nose before you begin.

2. Come into Proper Sitting Alignment with your eyes closed. Keep your mouth closed for the entire sequence.

3. Place your left hand on your belly and bring your right hand under your nose with the palm facing down so that you can feel the air coming out of your nostrils.

4. Inhale and then exhale forcefully (as though you are trying to expel a bug from your nose). Feel your belly sharply and simultaneously move in toward the spine as you do this.

5. Allow your inhalation to come spontaneously without forcing it.

6. Repeat steps 4 and 5 (one round) slowly, and then begin to build speed. Focus only on the forceful exhalations as you create a distinct rhythm.

7. Continue for up to fifty rounds.

8. Finally, inhale deeply and then exhale through the mouth with a sigh, "Aah."

9. Lower your arms into your lap and sit in stillness for several moments. Notice the effects of this powerful energizing breath.

Through yoga, I have learned how to find the energy that is hiding within me, waiting to be found.

— HANAN ABBASSI, YOGA STUDENT

When to avoid this posture The Breath of Fire is not recommended for people with epilepsy, for pregnant or menstruating women, or for those with ear infections, glaucoma, high blood pressure, or heart problems.

Yoga Tip In Sanskrit, this breath is known as a skull cleanser. It involves a series of rapid exhalations followed by passive inhalations. The staccato action causes a rocking motion in the cerebrospinal fluid that surrounds the brain. The pumping of the exhalations is like giving your brain an internal massage. Use it during strenuous postures to enhance your endurance level. It is *not* to be confused with hyperventilation. If you begin to hyperventilate or feel lightheaded, stop immediately and allow your breath to normalize. Proceed slowly, starting with ten rounds. Avoid doing more than fifty rounds of this powerful breath.

BODY OF ENERGY

*T*his experience was inspired by David Gershon and Gail Straub. What is your Energy level on a typical day? Is it generally high, low, or somewhere in the middle? The life force is unlimited; we rarely tap into our Energy potential.

Let's begin:

1. Come into your favorite version of the Corpse Pose with your eyes closed.

2. Take several long, deep, soothing breaths. Feel your body sinking down into the comfort of the ground beneath you.

3. Imagine that you are lying in the sun. This sun cannot burn or hurt you. Rather, it can only heal and bathe you in its powerful Energy.

4. Feel the sun's rays shining down on you and surrounding your body with a radiating light that nourishes every cell.

5. Spend several minutes basking in these healing rays that warm and invigorate your being.

6. Once you are fully energized, in your mind's eye see yourself getting up. Imagine that you are so filled with Energy that it actually radiates out from your body.

7. You are vibrant, vital and alive. Watch and feel yourself experience any and all of the physical possibilities within you. See yourself dance, run, lift, stretch, and play with boundless Energy.

8. What does it feel like to be limitless in your abilities?

9. Now watch as your limitless endurance allows you to do all of the things that you want to do, for as long as you would like. See yourself making love for hours without fatigue, playing tag with your children all day, swimming from one island to another with outstanding stamina.

10. What does it feel like to have limitless endurance and stamina?

11. Feel the power and physical strength of your amazing body. Every fiber of your being is dynamically alive. Watch yourself easily pulling someone's car out of a snowbank, lifting the copy machine in your office and moving it to another part of the building, pulling a garbage truck down the road so that the garbage collectors can take a break.

12. What does it feel like to have incredible power and physical strength?

13. Note the perfect health of your body. See yourself clearly radiating this health. Notice others commenting on how healthy and vibrant you look. Feel deeply in each cell that you are the picture of health.

14. How does it feel to be in perfect health? Breathe it in.

15. Stay with these feelings and spend some time doing whatever you wish with this body that has amazing levels of endurance and stamina. Watch and feel what it is like to live in a powerful, strong, and healthy body.

16. Know that to the degree you can clearly picture yourself in this manner, you can manifest it as well. This Energy resides within you, perhaps not to leap tall buildings in a single bound, but to be in your body boldly, proudly, and with tremendous vigor.

17. When you feel complete, come back to lying in the warm, healing sun. Allow the rays to mirror your own radiance.

18. Know that you can return to this experience whenever you want, and gently begin to deepen your breath. Feel your body in contact with the ground beneath you.

19. Roll your body onto one side, hugging your knees toward your chest.

20. Bring your re-energized body into a seated position. Open your eyes when you are ready. You may wish to write about or draw this experience. Use the sun as a daily reminder of your inner Energy.

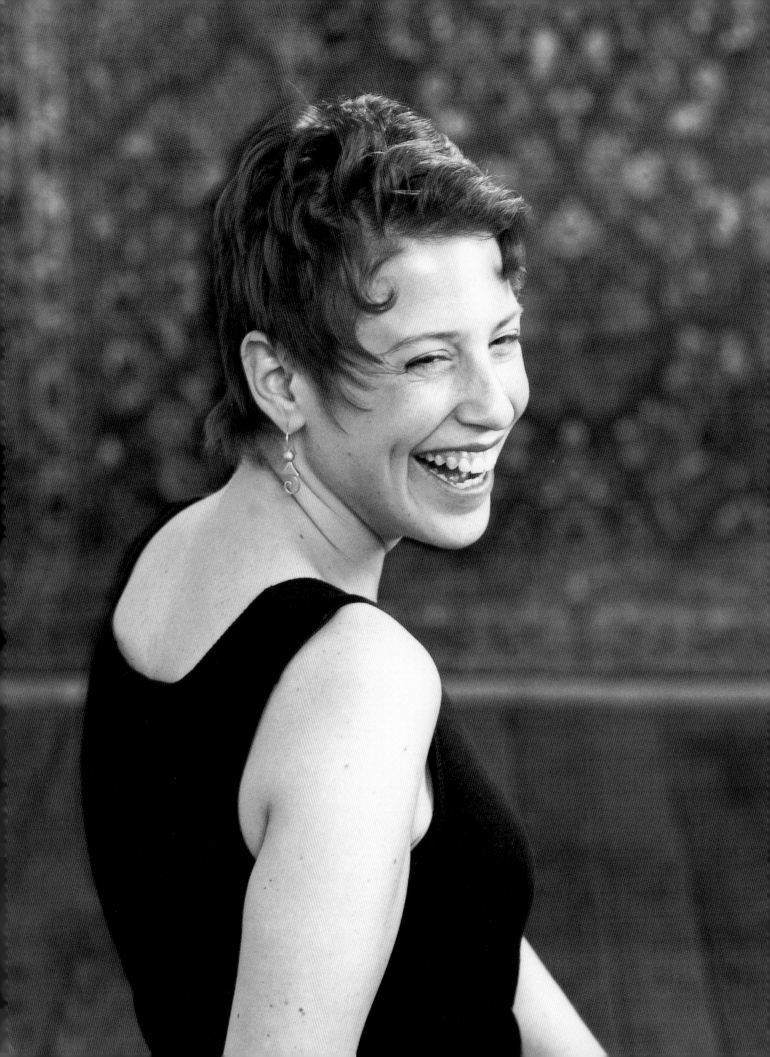

PLAYFULNESS

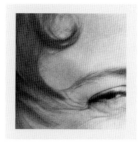

*T*hink back on playful moments you had as a child. Can you recall dressing up for Halloween, licking the spoon from a cookie mix, or being sprayed by a hose in the summertime? What was your inner experience at these treasured moments? These memories are viscerally stored as authentic feelings of being carefree, totally connected to the moment, and of tremendous and limitless happiness.

To let go of worrying who is watching or if you are "doing it right" is not always easy. When you choose not to be playful, it is often because you are concerned about what *they* will think. Your Inner Rules and Judgment Committee might be extremely loud.

Like any skill or attitude you wish to develop, Playfulness requires consistent attention and practice. It's far too easy to get sidetracked into seriousness, attached to thoughts and attitudes, or always having to be right. The good news is that Playfulness is habit forming and fosters spiritual joy in your life.

As adults, we can be child*like,* which is altogether different from child*ish.* Playfulness can extend into the workplace, the bedroom, and your daily routine. Bring a yo-yo to the office and try your hand at it during a break. Laugh together when you make love. Listen to fun, upbeat music next time you do the dishes. Have a talk with your Inner Rules and Judgment Committee. Maybe they want to have fun, too, but don't know how.

Creativity reconnects us to the world of inner play. To a child, a simple stone can become a musical instrument, a character in a play, or an ingredient in mud soup. Play with paint, words, and sounds to create your own art, stories, and music.

Living a spiritual path means cultivating opportunities to celebrate the magic and miracle of this gift called Life. Most traditions invite their communities to sing and dance for the love of the higher good. Gospel singing is an exhilarating and

The soul of one who loves god always swims in joy, always keeps holiday,
and is always in the mood for singing.

—SAINT JOHN OF THE CROSS

*Be merry, really merry. The life of a true Christian should be a perpetual jubilee,
a prelude to the festival of eternity.*

—THEOPHANE VENARD

engaging way to praise the Lord. Who wouldn't want to go to church with that joyous, energizing music to look forward to? Sufis twirl and Hasidic Jews dance themselves into ecstasy.

Humor and satire have played a historical role in many religious traditions. Clowns, holy fools, and silly plays were once popular means to unravel the rigidity and seriousness of church members. Before the Protestant Reformation, even priests and bishops performed acts of buffoonery, making fun of the strict laws of the church.

Comedy may seem blasphemous in the context of religion. When used correctly, however, it can stir up a sense of the sacred. When people laugh together by watching role reversals, tricksters, or some other religious incongruity, they come together as a community. Establishing reverence for levity can unite people in an integral way.

Many spiritual masters use humorous stories to convey their messages. His Holiness the Dalai Lama carries the tragic and heavy weight of the Tibetan people, yet he is delightfully playful and lighthearted. Some Zen instructors teach smiling meditations to create more spaciousness in the mind. And they don't call Him the Laughing Buddha for nothing! The word *guru* literally means "one who brings you from darkness into light." My favorite

definition is to simply spell the word out loud: G-U-R-U.

In your yoga practice, maintain a lighthearted approach. Create space for levity. Allow the sacred movements to draw you into festivity. Explore the movements of your body with childlike wonder. Let go of the preoccupation with perfection. Spend time recalling cosmic jokes and use them to strengthen your playful purpose. Let your attempts to balance, flex, and twist be grist for the mill of self-enjoyment. And don't forget one of the most important postures of all—turning up the corners of your mouth.

Postures for Playfulness While all of the postures in this book should be practiced with a lighthearted attitude, Shake Off, Peanut Butter Jar, The Lion, Spinal Rocking, and the Half-Circle are inherently playful. They are sure to tickle your funny bone while they benefit your body.

Breathing Lesson for Playfulness You will find it difficult to wear a sour face when you experience the Breath of Joy. Practice this breath and you'll feel jovial, enthusiastic, and rejuvenated!

Visualization for Playfulness "Look Again!" switches your mental channel from a soap opera to a sitcom. Change your "Ooh-no's" to "Aaa-ha's," or better yet, "Ha-ha's."

Over the years, I've had many executives come to me and say with pride: "Boy, last year I worked so hard that I didn't take any vacation." It's actually nothing to be proud of. I always feel like responding, "You dummy. You mean to tell me that you can take responsibility for an $80 million project and you can't plan two weeks out of the year to go off with your family and have some fun?"

—LEE IACOCCA FROM *IACOCCA: AN AUTOBIOGRAPHY*

YOGA STORY FOR PLAYFULNESS: NATESHVAR KEN SCOTT

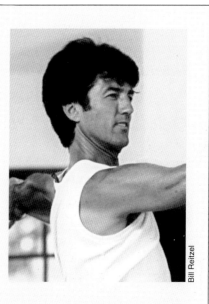

Yoga is fun. Anyone not convinced of that has yet to meet Nateshvar. He is a wizard in the art of teaching yoga in a playful way. From the age of four, gymnastics was his yoga. As an adult, he worked as an acrobat/stuntman for a dance company and later became a dancer in the troupe. Dance evolved into aerobics. His search for a playful venue for his creativity led him to yoga. He is the founder of ContactYoga™ and JoyYoga. When asked about Playfulness, he replied:

Let's play with that a little bit!

For me, yoga is an invitation to play. When I do the Cobra, I feel the energy of the snake as I slither and slide across the floor on my belly. We must allow ourselves imagination and a full range of expressiveness. What would it feel like to really be the Lion? What level of freedom and depth of sight would I experience if I were an Eagle? There's nothing I enjoy more than understanding, on a kinesthetic level, the nature of all that inhabits God's kingdom. I am certain that God must be love, laughter, harmony, peace, and an integration of all beings.

One of our greatest means of expression is through our voices. I like to make sounds, moans, roars, cries, and belly laughs when I move through the postures—anything goes! When we allow ourselves the full range of animation—through sound, movement, feeling—we become vehicles for joy. Yoga's a playful festival of tuning into the energy of the various animals and parts of nature that it is based on.

I create stories for my students to enact through yoga. If the story is about a tree on a mountain with an eagle flying above, my students become these elements. Sometimes I feel like a little elf, telling a magical story and watching the characters (my students) come to life. When yoga is made playful, our fear and self-consciousness fall away; we have permission to be in our bodies.

Joy is a byproduct of Playfulness. It's like an adrenaline rush that feeds the organs of the body differently than if we are trying to attain the postures through hard work and discipline. It's not that hard work and discipline aren't necessary, but that by being spontaneous and doing what feels joyful, we transcend our egos and enter an open-hearted space.

The best way to come to joy is through jokes and laughter.

—RABBI NACHMAN OF BRATSLOV

SHAKE OFF

Body Benefits:

➤ Improves circulation and generates heat

➤ Releases tension

➤ Lubricates joints

➤ Brings blood to extremities

➤ Energizes entire system

When to avoid this posture Do not practice Shake Off if you have joint disease. Proceed slowly and with caution if you are pregnant.

Yoga Tip Children are the best role models for developing the Spiritual Muscle of Playfulness. Join them as they twirl around in circles, skip along the sidewalk, and take a ride down the slide. Laughter, especially whole-body laughter, is good medicine. Four-year-olds laugh an average of four hundred times a day, while adults are lucky if they chuckle ten times! Visit your closest three-or four-year-old for some play therapy and try Shake-Off. They'll love it!

Let's begin:

1. Assume Proper Standing Alignment.

2. Imagine that you accidentally stepped in a pile of dog poop with your right foot. Begin to shake that foot furiously as if to rid yourself of the mess.

3. As you do this, you realize that the right foot was not the only one with bad luck. You must now switch feet and shake the mess off your left foot.

4. Now that your feet are cleaned off, shift your focus to that moment when you step out of the shower. Take an imaginary towel behind you, one end in each hand, and begin to wipe your behind dry. Come on. Everyone does it. Swing your hips from side to side.

5. With your backside dried off, move your awareness into your hands and arms. You see a swarm of fleas around them. Wave your hands and arms around furiously to shoo them all away. Flick your wrists.

6. Begin to notice your shoulders. Shimmy them front and back like a jazz dancer.

7. Now bring your attention to your head. Shake your head side to side as if to say "No way!"

8. Then bounce it up and down with a big "YES!"

9. Now that you're "all shook up," go back to the beginning and shake everything at once: your feet, legs, buttocks and hips, arms and hands, shoulders, and head. Let loose! Go crazy! Act like you're losing your mind—in a pleasant way. Continue for ten seconds.

10. To complete, inhale as you raise your hands overhead. Hold them there for a few seconds as if you are waiting to hear something very important.

11. In slow motion, exhale and allow your arms to circle down to your sides, noticing every inch of the release. Did you release more than just your arms? What about worry, stress, and seriousness?

12. Stand for a moment in Proper Standing Alignment and take several deep breaths.

What did the yogi say when he walked into the pizza parlor?
"Make me one with everything."

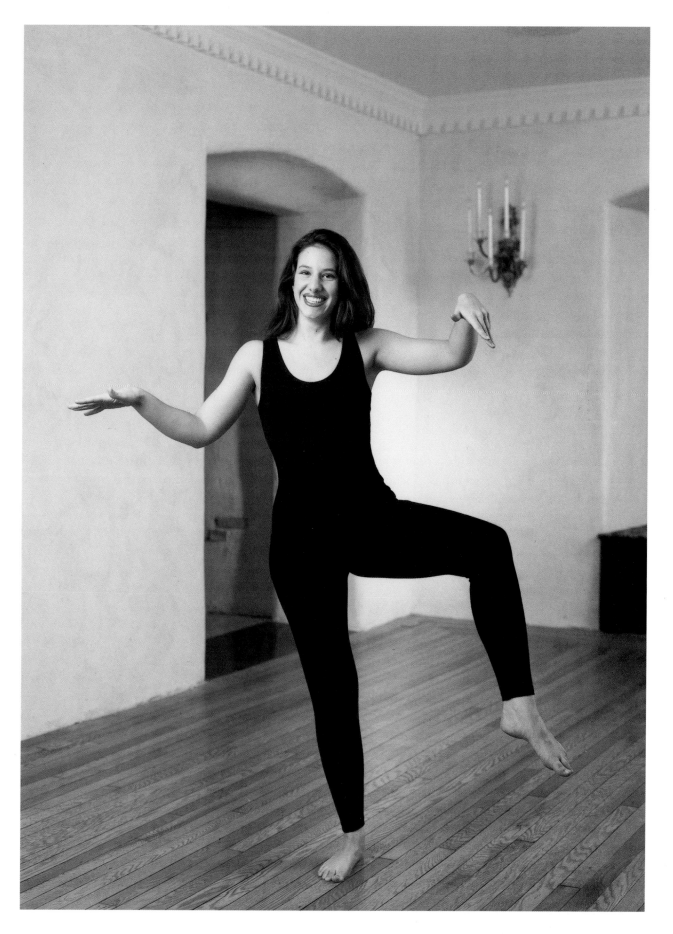

PEANUT BUTTER JAR

Body Benefits:

➤ Rotates, warms, and flexes spine

➤ Improves breathing

➤ Activates peristalsis (digestion) and relieves constipation

➤ Increases circulation

➤ Brings heat to body

➤ Brings fresh oxygen to musculoskeletal system

➤ Opens pelvis

➤ Lubricates hip joints and shoulder girdle

Let's begin:

1. Begin in the Table position. You will remain on your hands and knees throughout this experience.

2. Pretend that you are inside a giant peanut butter jar that is almost empty. Your job is to scoop out the remains of the peanut butter *with your body*.

Yoga Tip Just as not every part of your life needs to be structured, not every part of your yoga practice must be a formal exercise. Allow your inner movements to come into *play*. Be creative and feel every part of your body delight in its own process of unfolding. Immerse yourself in a pool of joy as you nurture yourself in authentic movement.

3. Use your hips, buttocks, shoulders, head, and the sides of your torso to clean out the jar. Be creative and have fun!

4. The Peanut Butter Jar can be like a combination of the Six Movements of the Spine.

5. Try to match the pattern of your breath with the pattern of the movements that you are creating.

6. Let your movements be a surprise, a spontaneous improvisation.

7. When you have scooped all the peanut butter out of the jar, remain in the Table position for a moment. Check in and become aware of how you are feeling.

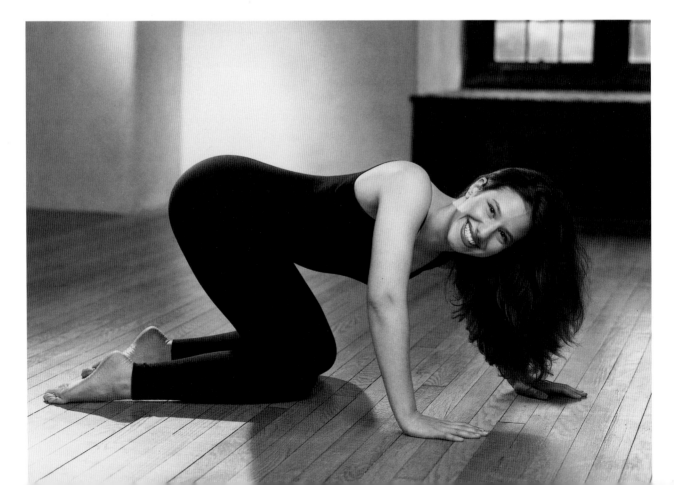

LION

> *Yoga Tip* In some cultures, the tongue is a symbol of power. In our culture, we eat and talk with the tongue, but rarely exercise it. This is a great pose with a partner or in a circle with a group. (It's even sillier when you wear funny glasses!) Kids love this pose and so will you. You may want to practice facing a mirror, but don't try this on the subway!

Body Benefits:

➤ Increases circulation to tongue, face, neck, and throat

➤ Helps to alleviate a sore throat

➤ Strengthens voice and facial muscles

➤ Improves complexion, bad breath

➤ Helps relieve depression

➤ Recommended to help cure stammering

Let's begin:

1. Sit on your heels or in Proper Sitting Alignment.

2. Rest your hands on your knees with your fingers spread apart.

3. Pretend you are a fierce, powerful lion. Take a deep breath through your nose as you lengthen your spine.

4. Lean forward slightly and exhale through your mouth as long as you can with a roaring "Aaah." Extend your tongue out, raise your fingers off your knees and shape them into stiff claws. Open your eyes and mouth wide.

5. When you run out of breath, close your mouth, relax your eyes and fingers, and inhale through your nose. Sit back on your heels once again.

6. Repeat steps 2–5 several times.

7. When complete, sit quietly for a moment and notice your inner experience.

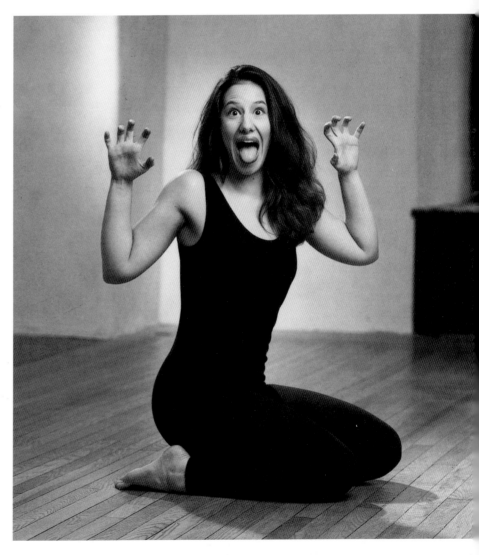

If all business meetings began with everyone sitting around a conference table doing the Lion, the world would be a friendlier place.

—JULIAROSE LOFFREDO, YOGA STUDENT

HALF-CIRCLE

Body Benefits:

➤ Energizes and decongests nervous system

➤ Increases flexibility in spine

➤ Expands lung capacity and improves respiration

➤ Provides kidneys with fresh blood supply

➤ Tones legs, buttocks, back, shoulders, arms, and wrists

➤ Improves circulation and heats body

When to avoid this posture Do not practice the Half-Circle if you have a hernia.

Yoga Tip To deepen the stretch, imagine that a hundred dollar bill or a winning lottery ticket is just out of reach. You'll be surprised at how much farther you can go. Allen Klein, "jollitologist" and author of *The Healing Power of Humor*, recommends replacing stressful events with fun activities. If you are stuck in a traffic jam, he suggests blowing soap bubbles out the window for all to enjoy. Try this: Think about how you would feel with a huge, toothy grin on your face. Now— do it. Go ahead! C'mon, make it even sillier. How does it feel? It's difficult to worry when you are having fun.

The mystic uses laughter and a holy shamelessness as one of his or her most powerful weapons. People who've realized their divine identity know that they are entirely blessed by God in all their silliness and frivolity, and this releases them into the dance of humor, which heals and releases everyone around them.

—ANDREW HARVEY,

FROM *DIALOGUES WITH A MODERN MYSTIC*

Let's begin:

1. Start in a seated position with your legs spread apart. Bend the right knee and bring the right foot in towards your groin.

2. Use the right hand for support on the floor beside your right hip. Maintain a lengthened spine.

3. Raise your left hand overhead. Lift the pelvis up off the floor. You are now carrying the weight of your body on the right hand and the right shin.

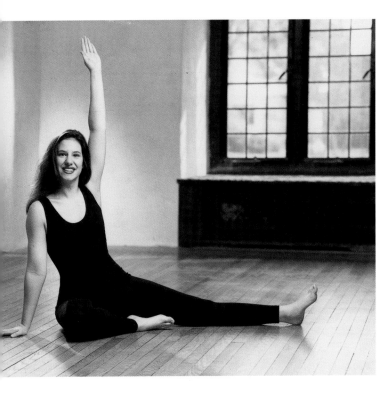

4. Extend the left arm over to the right as if you are reaching for something in the air. Keep the left leg straight with only the left toes on the ground.

5. As the left toes press into the floor, you will feel a deep stretch across the entire left side of the body. Breathe deeply.

6. To release, slide the left leg out along the ground and lower the buttocks back to the floor. Take a deep breath. As you exhale, lower the left arm.

7. Repeat steps 1–6 on the opposite side.

8. When you have completed both sides, sit for a moment and check in with yourself.

CREATE YOUR OWN POSTURE FOR PLAYFULNESS

Let's begin:

1. Practice the formal postures before creating your own.

2. Begin in any position that feels comfortable, eyes closed. Take several deep breaths while the corners of your mouth turn upward.

3. Bring to mind an animal, cartoon character, clown, or any other funny being that you choose. Imitate its movements and expressions. For instance, if it's a raccoon, begin to crawl around as you imagine this creature would. If it's a clown, imagine yourself wearing a big red nose and green hair, and walk bowlegged.

4. Start to get goofy now. Play silly songs or make the fun noises that your favorite comic character makes.

5. Allow your body to move in any way that feels light and playful.

6. When you find a position that you keep returning to or want to hold, stop moving. Stay here and breathe, exploring the micromovements that help lighten this playful pose.

7. Name your posture and make a note of how you feel in it. Create a statement that confirms your commitment to Playfulness. Draw a picture of your posture or write about how it felt to be the King or Queen of Silly.

BREATH OF JOY

Body Benefits:

➤ Invigorates body

➤ Clears mind

➤ Alleviates sadness and mild depression

➤ Rids lungs of stale air

➤ Stimulates digestion

➤ Filters pollutants

When to avoid this exercise If you have uncontrolled high blood pressure or a history of heart disease or stroke, or if you are pregnant, do not practice the Breath of Joy.

Breathing Tip In this exercise, you will be moving your arms like an orchestra conductor. This is your chance to star in your own musical production. Practice slowly at first. Let yourself work up to a dramatic and extravagant finale. Try the Breath of Joy when you are experiencing the 3 P.M. slump or when you feel a little down.

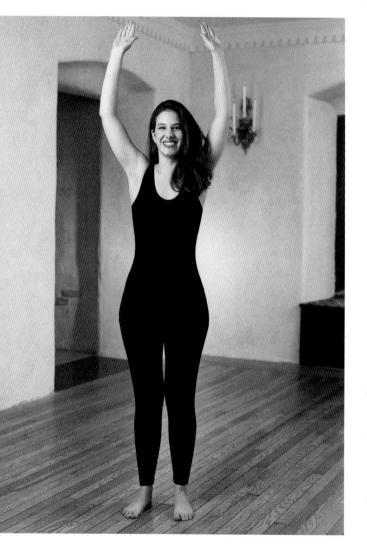

Angels fly because they take themselves lightly.
— G. K. CHESTERTON

Let's begin:

1. Start in Proper Standing Alignment.

2. Close the mouth. Inhale through the nose with a quick sniff as you sweep your arms up in front of you until they are overhead.

3. Inhale a second quick sniff through your nose as you swing the arms out to your sides.

4. Inhale a third quick sniff through your nose as you bring your arms back overhead (the way they were in step 2).

5. Now *exhale* through your mouth with a "Ha!" as you swing the arms down in a loose sweeping motion. Bend at the waist and knees so that your head and torso hang down toward the floor. Release the head and relax the neck muscles (as if you were in the Rag Doll).

6. Inhale through the nose as you rebound swinging the arms overhead and come back to standing.

7. Steps 2–6 are performed in a flowing manner without stopping. Repeat these steps four or five times with outrageous embellishment.

8. To finish, let your arms return to your sides in Proper Standing Alignment with your eyes closed.

9. Check in and notice any sensations in your body. Can you feel your heart beating? The blood rushing? Do you feel more awake and zany?

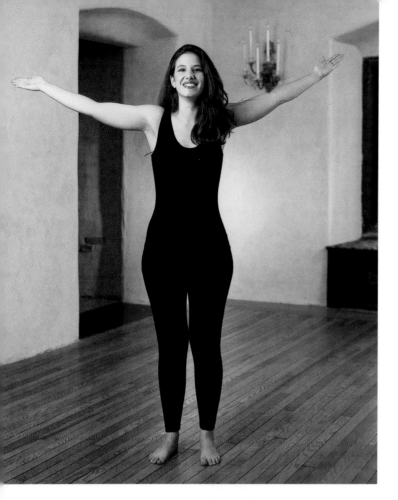

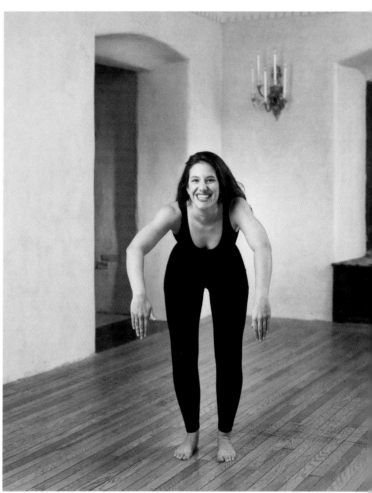

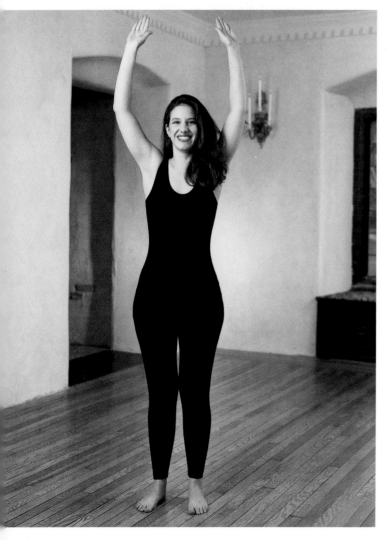

SPINAL ROCKING

Body Benefits:

- ➤ Improves spinal flexibility
- ➤ Massages and lengthens back
- ➤ Stimulates thyroid functioning
- ➤ Rejuvenates entire system
- ➤ Improves circulation
- ➤ Brings heat into body

Let's begin:

1. Sit on your buttocks with your legs in front of you. Bend your knees and hug them toward your chest. Your feet are flat on the floor.

2. Clasp your hands behind your knees or just below the front of the knees.

3. Bring your chin toward your chest.

4. Begin to rock backwards, rolling along the right side of the spine. Roll back up along the left side. Do not roll directly on the spine.

5. Be playful as you rock and roll around. Find as many different ways to roll around as you can.

6. When you are done, roll yourself up to a comfortable seated position, close your eyes, and check in.

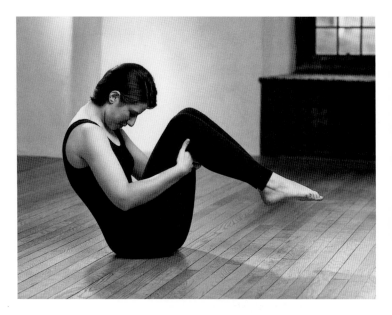

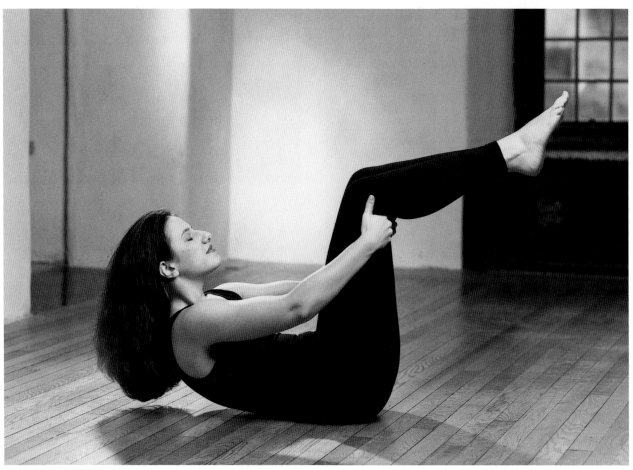

When to avoid this posture Do not practice Spinal Rocking if you are pregnant or have any neck or spinal ailments. Avoid this pose if you have glaucoma, detached retina, or uncontrolled high blood pressure.

Yoga Tip Rocking is as soothing as it is fun. Children are rocked to sleep; they play on rocking horses and rock and roll down hills. Pretend you are in kindergarten as you rock. Spinal Rocking is the quintessence of a pure and frolicsome spirit.

LOOK AGAIN!

Yoga Tip People of other cultures view some of the events we consider solemn with a sense of lightheartedness. Even death is played with in some traditions. For example, *Banda* is a traditional Haitian funeral dance. Because they see dying as a transformation, Haitians celebrate the fact that someone is passing through the door of death. They use fun costumes and cigars to laugh at death. See how many different ways you can reinterpret your own current episodes in life's many dilemmas.

Let's begin:

1. Come into the Corpse Pose.

2. Take five or more deep breaths until you feel relaxed and centered.

3. Think of a recent event that made you feel uncomfortable, angry, or unsettled.

4. In your imagination, replay the scene from beginning to end as if you were watching a play in your mind.

5. Recall who was with you, where you were, and what preceded the event.

6. What was the weather like? Could you hear any sounds? Smell any scents?

7. Most importantly, notice how you felt during the time that this scene took place.

8. Once you have replayed the entire scene, imagine a stage curtain closing on it.

9. Take several deep breaths to help you clear the scene from your emotional memory.

10. Now, replay the same act in your mind, but this time *change* all of the parts you did not like. For example, let's say that your scenario involved your boss yelling at you. She was right in your face with breath that could stun a monkey. Instead, imagine that your boss, whose breath smells of lilac bushes, is complimenting you on all your fine deeds and performance. Or exaggerate and make it silly. Visualize your boss throwing twenty dollar bills at you screaming, "Here, your salary is too small! Take my paycheck." It doesn't have to make sense. In fact, it shouldn't.

11. You are rewriting a tragedy or drama into a comedy, perhaps even a musical.

12. Go through the entire scene, noticing how you feel with your custom alterations.

13. Of course you have not changed the situation in reality, but you have opened your mind to alternative ways of thinking about the situation. You may have gained some levity and can return to real life with a new perspective and a clearer outlook.

14. Remain on your back for several minutes enjoying the comic relief before returning to your day more refreshed, energized, and open-minded.

15. In slow motion, deepen your breath and roll over on one side. Hug your knees into fetal position.

16. When you are ready, bring yourself and your sense of humor back with you into a comfortable seated position. Allow your eyes to open slowly.

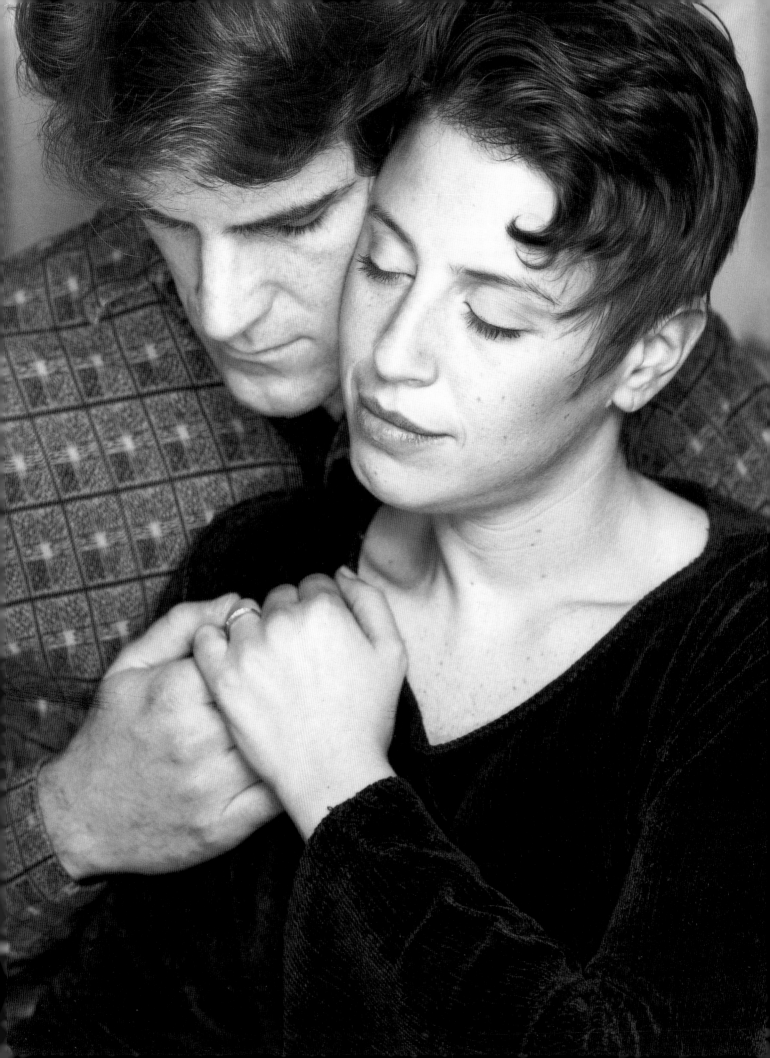

CONNECTEDNESS

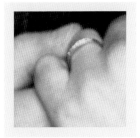

The quality of our relationships—with ourselves, others, and the world around us— determines the quality of our lives. To the degree that we feel connected, we will also feel that our life has meaning. Knowing that you are connected to me and that I am connected to you gives both our lives more purpose.

The need to belong starts at infancy and continues throughout life. Studies show that both human and animal babies need to feel connected. One of the most profound ways that new beings get this need met is through touch. Premature babies and animal newborns grow and develop faster with loving physical attention. Older children also need contact on many levels as their world expands through play and school.

Adults join groups of all kinds to feel connected to others. Fraternal, religious, political, volunteer, and countless other groups are paths to connection. The more fragmented our society becomes, the more we crave community. Programs like the Twelve Steps help redefine community into a framework that supports our whole selves and provide order and values to our sometimes chaotic lives.

Many cultures honor their ancestors and believe that their spirits are ever present, helping to guide them. Modern society often scoffs this off as primitive, but much of who we are is a result of who we came from. Denying our heritage cuts us off from this rich source of sustenance. At the other

end of the spectrum, children and visionaries show us the possibilities of future connections. Linking ourselves to the past and the future grounds us in the present.

Nearly every religious tradition is founded on the principle of Connectedness to a spiritual presence. Sufis pray *"Astaghfiru'llah"* or "I ask forgiveness of God"—forgiveness for being separate. All of the major religions have either a sacred written text of prayers or an oral tradition of stories linking generation after generation to their heritage. Within these authoritative writings or narratives are the holy laws that unite the people to each other and to a higher power.

If your body is the temple for your spirit and the kingdom of heaven exists within the consciousness of your thoughts, it is of little importance whether you are Christian, Muslim, Buddhist, or a member of any other belief system. Yoga can help you deepen your connection to yourself, your beliefs, your spirit, and other people.

Shouldn't we congregate as a race of human beings? Let us transcend our differences in order to see our commonalties. There are many paths to the

177

sacred. If it is inner transformation we are seeking, then what does the external form matter? When whatever we do is done with reverence, our lives are a delightful journey toward connection.

Connectedness is not only fulfilling but necessary for survival. According to author Joan Borysenko, there are two essential steps to healing. One is high self-esteem and the other is a strong support group. Without connection to others, people are at higher risk for heart disease. Isolation can lead to illness.

Yoga is a Sanskrit word meaning "union" or "yoke" or "to harness together." In electronics, a yoke is a piece of magnetic material that permanently connects two or more magnets. In human terms, yoga helps magnetize us to that which most nourishes our spirits.

One of the most joyful ways we can learn to connect is through partner yoga. Practicing yoga with a friend has many advantages. You'll be able to go more deeply into the poses with the help of another. You can hold difficult postures longer while learning to both give and receive support. And last but not least, it's fun! When you do yoga with a partner, you connect to yourself and another in a sacred way—sharing the essence of yoga.

When we experience communion—whether with a higher power, nature, other people, animals, or ourselves—we tap into life-sustaining and life-enhancing resources. These connections reverberate in our essence and comprise the ultimate treasures of our lives, the rich experience of oneness. As we integrate body, mind, and spirit through yoga, we become whole. Derived from the same root, being whole is our link to being both healthy and holy.

Postures for Connectedness You'll enjoy the See-Saw, Partner Pretzel Twist, and the Fountain with a friend, lover, or coworker. When done in partnership, you can go even deeper into the Perfect Gate and the Double Tree than you can on your own.

Breathing Lesson for Connectedness Unity Breath is a beautiful, relaxing, and profoundly sacred breath to do with another person.

Relaxation for Connectedness You may be surprised at the intimacy that develops from this simple hands-off massage technique called Invisible Touch.

LITTLE YOGIS: CONNECTING WITH KIDS THROUGH YOGA

*Y*oga is a great way to spend time together with your kids (or somebody else's) in an intimate and genuine way. Kids love to move and stretch their bodies, and they'll certainly appreciate the time together with you. If we all learned yoga growing up, who knows—maybe we'd all be enlightened by the fourth grade! Encouraging children to open and trust themselves and their bodies leads them to the world of possibilities. When doing yoga with little yogis, keep these guidelines in mind:

➤ Create a special ritual to begin and end your yoga time together. You might start with a symbolic bow to each other. You could end by sitting back to back, practicing Unity Breath together.

➤ Use sound. Roar when you do the Lion. Bark in the Dog. Play relaxing or energizing music depending upon your moods.

➤ Do partner postures gently and support their bodies as much as you can. Make up your own fun ways to be together, so that you also get to stretch.

➤ Add a few minutes of silence into your practice. Tell your little partners that all the parts of their bodies need a rest: eyes, voices, minds, arms, and legs. Have a special yoga bell that one of you rings when silent time is over.

➤ Be encouraging! Tell them what great yoga masters they are. Remember that yoga is

When Unity is established within yourself, everything is related, the whole universe becomes one vast tree of life; once we enter the life of that tree we can proceed to any point on its branches.

—N. SRI RAM

not competitive. Whatever they do is fabulous.

➤ Ask them what their favorite posture is and do that one first. Invite them to add their own unique touch. In the Breath of Joy they can say their favorite foods three times when they are upright and call out the food they hate most as they sweep their arms down.

➤ Get into yoga from a child's viewpoint. In the Bridge, have them imagine water rushing under them. Ask them what it would be like to be a slithering Cobra with no arms and legs. In Standing Yoga Mudra, pretend you are bowing to the King and Queen of Sillyville.

➤ Let them lead you in any movements they want. Play follow the leader and take turns teaching every other posture.

➤ Talk about breathing. Invite them to put their hands on their bellies and feel them move like a balloon. Have them put their hands under their nostrils to notice which one the air is coming out of. Invite them to put their heads on your belly to feel the movement. Exhale as if blowing out birthday candles. Tell them their breath is the magic part of them that stays with them throughout their whole lives so they can do all the things they want to do.

➤ Try practicing yoga as a family or when the kids have friends over. Sit in a circle facing each other and do Spinal Rocking. Join hands in a circle and create movements without letting go of your hands. Notice whose head or whose rear end bobs up at the same time as yours. Put your feet in the middle of the circle and tickle each others toes, playing footsies.

➤ Lead them in a minirelaxation. Let them close their eyes and pretend they are having a dream or are watching a movie inside their heads.

➤ Practice yoga outdoors. Use your imagination and encourage them to use theirs. Have them pretend they are Mountains and Trees.

➤ Make up your own postures. Find ways to move parts of the body you don't normally stretch. How can you move your elbow, your toes, your eyebrows? You might want to use a mirror for some laughs.

➤ Help them develop concentration skills by allowing them to choose and look at one special spot for the whole time they hold a posture. Tell them how eagles and other animals keep their focus on one thing and that they can too!

➤ Keep it safe. Use pillows and soft surroundings so you are both protected.

➤ Vary the movements so they can get a full range of experiences. Do Shake Off to help make use of their energy. Practice some quiet postures like the Hero and whisper when you lead it.

➤ Count together as you hold the posture for as long as they can comfortably do it. Never get into any kind of pain or discomfort. Encourage kids to enjoy being in their bodies.

➤ Tell them the benefits of yoga. Explain that yoga helps people stay strong and healthy, do well in school, and feel great!

When human beings lose their connection to nature, to heaven and earth, then they do not know how to nurture their environment or how to rule their world—which is saying the same thing. Human beings destroy their ecology at the same time that they destroy one another. From that perspective, healing our society goes hand in hand with healing our personal, elemental connection with the phenomenal world.

—CHÖGYAM TRUNGPA

YOGA STORY FOR CONNECTEDNESS: DAVID GERSHON AND GAIL STRAUB

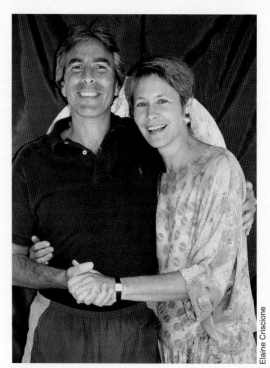

Elaine Criscione

David Gershon and Gail Straub have devoted their lives to healing the lack of Connectedness on both individual and planetary levels. They are mythic characters and large-scale masters in the Yoga of Service. In addition to leading their world-popular Empowerment Workshops, Grace Training, and Fire in the Soul, they have masterminded international events such as The First Earth Run. This commemorated the United Nations Year of Peace, where a torch was passed among forty-five heads of state in sixty-two countries, symbolizing the possibility for hope in the world. Over twenty-five million people participated. David developed the Global Action Plan (GAP) for the Earth, which has received widespread international recognition as a method to help create a sustainable future.

Author: You are both deeply dedicated to nature as a primary way to connect to the world of spirit. How did that develop for you?

Gail: The time in my life when I felt I most belonged was during my childhood. I have always loved the natural world. I can remember how I loved being on the Earth. My sister and I were little tomboys, little monkeys. We climbed every tree in the neighborhood and had a special route around a brook in our backyard called "the pancake run." The physical connection I had to my little backyard world has been my window to the global world. My early love affair with the Earth led me to my life's mission.

David: My growing up in suburbia was different from Gail's experience. I was attracted to the outdoor world but I didn't have the same kind of opportunities. I felt like there was a hole in me. Later on in college I heard the beauty of nature calling me. It allowed me to connect to myself in a healing and soothing way. My GAP work now explicitly brings an awareness to people that these sacred resources need to be stewarded more carefully. I encourage people to reconnect with the Earth as a way to become better stewards.

Gail: There's so much talk about loss of soul. Part of that loss is the desecration of the Earth and the misuse of its resources. We are disconnected because of the belief that more is better and that we can just keep taking. Our Earth is the large soul that we're all a part of. If we become more caring of the Earth, we have a direct connection to our spirit.

Author: In your Empowerment Workshops, you have people create their own physical postures as a way to connect to the beliefs they are trying to create. What is that like?

David: Our Empowerment work has a lot to do with people getting in touch with their unique visions. We have them create a physical movement or gesture that helps them embody that vision. Many people have told us that the most powerful and integrated way they feel their vision and really own it is through kinesthetic movement. So they create a vision, an affirmation, and a movement—all of which reinforce each other. They enact the posture as a ritual.

Gail: A woman in my Grace training was very introverted. Her feminine side was beautiful and well developed. She wanted to develop more of her masculine side. Despite her deep prayer life, she had never added any physical components to it. She developed a warrior stance that was very grounded. She even held a symbolic sword. It became a powerful part of her prayer life, and she felt stronger and more balanced.

Author: When I have had the pleasure of observing you teach, I notice that you each have your own teaching posture. David, you lead standing very tall with your hands in front of your hara, your energy center. Gail, your hands are often together in front of your heart.

David: Wow, that's really true. I hold a center from a place of power and groundedness. That's the place that I hold my beliefs: one, that anything is possible; and two, to go for the biggest dream you can conceive. Gail leads differently. She connects to people through her heart, which is her main center for teaching.

Author: We were speaking of visions earlier. The First Earth Run that you led carrying a torch around the Earth was a monumental vision. It connected people in a way that transcended their differences.

David: Yes. We found that using the universal symbol of fire as our common spirit, raising money for children and the future, caring for the Earth, and wanting to create a more peaceful world were all transcendent ideas. Because it was a spiritual event, we were able to create openings that wouldn't otherwise be possible. The vision was larger than the differences, and it connected us all to something even larger. That kind of massive global ritual touches something very primal and deep inside of people. Many countries came together in a powerful way: north and south Ireland, an Arab and Jewish child, the Nicaraguan government and the Contras all passed the torch to each other.

Author: On another level, we all feel disconnected at certain periods of our lives. At what times do you feel that way and how do you reconnect?

Gail: It's a matter of how we ride the periods of boredom and disconnection. It helps me to know that this is a normal part of a dedicated spiritual path. We all want it to be smooth, without ups and downs. At moments when there is a crisis in faith, we need to remember that life has a way of testing our connection. If we know that the tests are part of the journey, we can get through them.

David: When I feel disconnected, I engage in something uplifting, something that helps me to feel very alive. When I feel alive, I feel connected. I consistently take care of my body and meditate, so my bank account is full. Then when I need to draw upon it, I can take out some of what I've built up.

Gail: The strongest thing that I do to reconnect is my prayer and meditation practice. We feed ourselves spiritually by entering a small meditation room we built onto our house. We invite others into this space as well. It's such a nourishing place to go when we're troubled.

David: I go to our meditation room when I want to feel connected. I conjure up an image of a beautiful place filled with luminous light and love. When I enter that, I feel oneness, connection with the universe and with all existence. This helps me embrace life's possibilities and hold a positive charge.

Author: You do a lot together as a couple, you often work together, and you share a common purpose. How does your connection to each other help you serve your larger goals?

Gail: We both feel tremendously blessed to have found our soul friend, or *anam cara*, as it is called in the Celtic tradition. We get a great deal of satisfaction working alone and observing each other's work. We've also learned a lot from working together. It would be easy to be consumed by the passion of service, but we also have a deep respect for our marriage. We don't take each other for granted. We take retreats throughout the year to renew the love and bond we have and to nurture our own connection.

See-Saw

Body Benefits:

➤ Tones, stretches, and lengthens spine and backs of legs

➤ Improves digestion and relieves constipation

➤ Stimulates pancreas, liver, gallbladder, spleen, urinary bladder, and gonads

➤ Increases circulation, especially in pelvic region

➤ Helps regulate menstrual irregularities

➤ Helps irrigate kidneys

When to avoid this posture Practice with caution if you suffer from sciatica or have stiff, weak back muscles.

Yoga Tip Be aware of whether you prefer to give or take in each stretch. Notice the ever-changing shift between giving and receiving in any relationship. In this and all of the partner postures, be sure to communicate with each other about how you are feeling: Is a stretch too much, not enough, or just right?

Let's begin:

1. Come into a seated position facing your partner.

2. Both partners: separate your outstretched legs as far as you comfortably can, touching each other's toes, ankles, or calves. Your connected legs will form a diamond.

3. Reach out to clasp hands or fingers. If possible, one partner can grab the other partner's wrists with palms down, the other with palms up. You may need to bend your knees slightly in order to touch.

4. Begin a gentle swaying motion back and forth; one partner is leaning back slightly while the other is drawn forward.

5. Be sure to breathe during the movement. You may want to develop a breathing pattern where you exhale while leaning forward, and then inhale while leaning back, or vice-versa.

6. Be playful while respecting each other's needs, differences, and limitations.

7. To complete, come back to center, and slowly separate hands. Bring your legs back together.

8. With your eyes closed, sit back-to-back in Proper Sitting Alignment for a few moments, connecting with each other's breath.

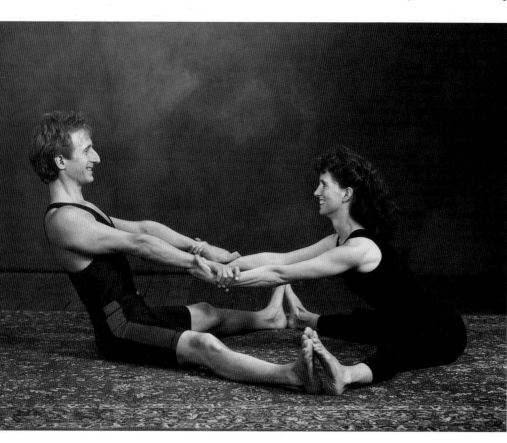

UNITY BREATH

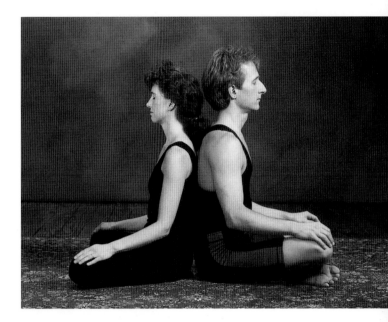

> **Yoga Tip** All sentient beings share the same air. In this experience, *consciously* share the breath. In doing so, you can come together in the most elemental and supportive way. You may use this technique *between* each posture as a way to reconnect.

Let's begin:

1. Come into Proper Sitting Alignment back-to-back with your eyes closed. You can sit either cross-legged or with one or both legs out in front of you.

2. Imagine that your partner's back is a supportive wall. Feel your spines and backs connected. Notice where they connect and how it feels to you.

3. Focus first on your own breath. Be sure to breathe naturally and deeply. Note how each inhalation is naturally linked to every exhalation.

4. Start to notice the pattern of breath that you two create together. Are you inhaling at the same time? Do you exhale together? Without trying to change it, simply notice.

5. Sit together in silence for several moments simply observing your own breath and sensing your partner's.

6. Imagine that you are wearing an uninflated inner tube around your belly. As you breathe, you fill the inner tube not only in front of you, but also behind you (against your partner's back) and to the sides. As you exhale, the inner tube deflates back in toward your body.

7. Now begin to experiment. Try to inhale at the same time. Feel your backs pressing against each other's as you inhale. Sense the gentle retreat as you exhale. Begin to breathe in unison for a few minutes.

8. To switch gears, take a deep breath in and sigh it out. Repeat two more times.

9. Now breathe in a complementary way: as one inhales, the other exhales. Try to create long, gentle breaths. Allow one partner's inhalation to last the length of the others' exhalation. Imagine that you are one working (and breathing) unit. Continue for a few minutes.

10. Take a deep breath in and sigh it out. Repeat this twice more.

11. Go back to simply noticing the breath without trying to change it. Feel the union between you. Notice how this unity affects your thoughts and emotions.

12. Remain sitting quietly back-to-back for several more breaths.

13. Take another few deep breaths in and out with sighs. When you are ready, gently open your eyes. Turn around to make eye contact with your partner.

14. Share with each other the experience that you had, including difficulties, pleasures, or other areas of interest. Be sure to thank your partner!

No one spoke, yet we communicated somehow. We were connecting with each other at a different level.

— KATYA COSTA, YOGA STUDENT

FOUNTAIN

Body Benefits:

➤ Expands lung capacity

➤ Improves circulation

➤ Opens chest

➤ Stimulates thyroid gland

➤ Energizes and heats body

➤ Replenishes kidneys with fresh blood and oxygen

When to avoid this posture Move slowly into the Fountain if you have weak back muscles.

Yoga Tip Imagine your body is a fountain. The water springs out from your upper chest. Focus on lifting the sternum high rather than simply arching back. You can maintain this graceful lift with the support of your partner. When it's time for both of you to get the stretch, picture a glorious fountain bursting forth from your upper torsos.

Let's begin:

1. Start in Proper Sitting Alignment with your legs crossed, facing each other. Bring your knees as close together as possible.

2. Reach forward and grab wrists. One partner has palms down and the other palms up.

3. One of you acts as the supporting partner while the other is the arching partner, and then you switch. Supporting partner: lean back slightly and keep a steady grip. Arching partner: begin to lift up from the chest, extending your sternum toward the ceiling. As you do, lift your chin up, cradle your head back into your shoulders, and arch back slowly. Both partners lean away gently from one another.

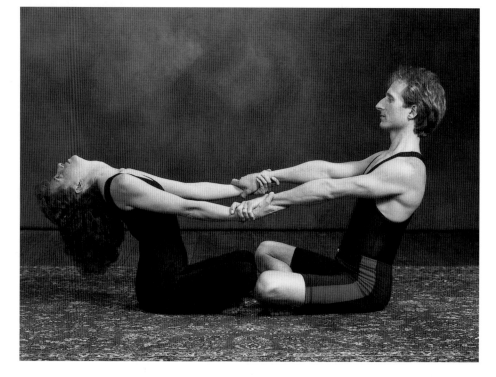

4. Arching partner: experiment with varying depths by descending slowly into the arch and hanging out at different points along the way.

5. Use each other's weight to support you. Keep breathing, and don't let go!

When I first started yoga, I was scared that it might conflict with my religious beliefs. I realize now that yoga can be practiced by anyone of any religion. As a matter of fact, it strengthened the relationship between me and God, because focusing and concentration during prayer helped me feel closer to him.

—RAZI ALIMAM, YOGA STUDENT

6. Arching partner: to come back up, first lift the head and then press down into your sitting bones, using the strength of your stomach muscles.

7. Allow the eyes to close for a moment. Feel the connection between your arms and then switch roles.

8. After you have each had the chance to arch, come back to center and go into the full Fountain by continuing to firmly clasp wrists. You may wish to switch the position of the hold so that the person whose palms were face down are now face up, and vice versa.

9. Both partners: lift out of the waist, press the chest toward the ceiling, and let your head fall back into the cradle of your shoulders.

10. Lean away from each other without letting go. Breathe deeply into the whole front side of your body, from the belly all the way up to the throat.

11. Communicate with each other by expressing your needs, limitations, and feelings.

12. When you are ready to come back up, squeeze your partner's wrists as a signal, or tell him or her you are complete. Lift your heads up first. Continue to lengthen up the spine. Use the abdominal muscles as you roll back up to sitting, lowering your arms.

13. With eyes closed, sit back-to-back in Proper Sitting Alignment for a few moments. Connect with each other's breath.

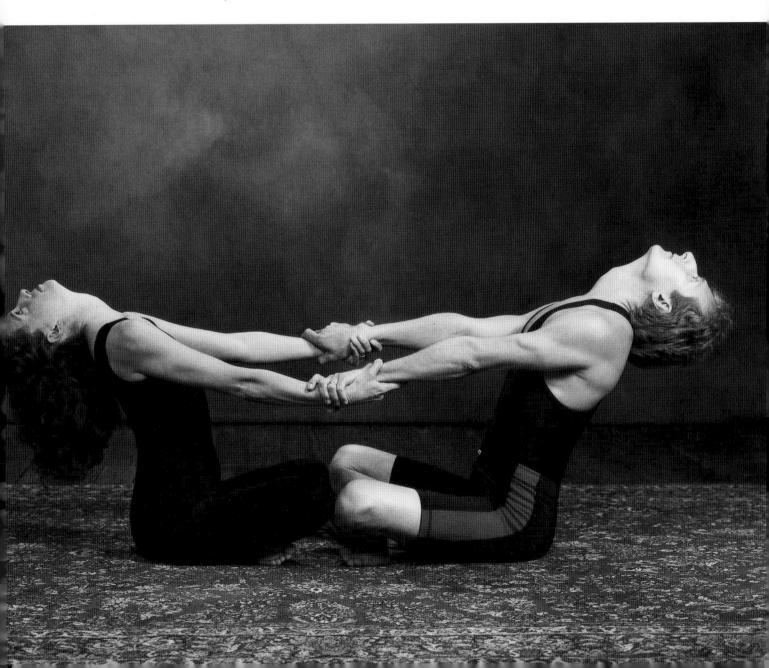

PERFECT GATE

Body Benefits:

➤ Energizes and decongests nervous system

➤ Increases flexibility in spine and pelvis

➤ Expands lung capacity and improves respiration

➤ Provides kidneys with fresh blood supply

➤ Tones legs, abdominals, buttocks, back, shoulders, and arms

➤ Improves circulation and heats body

Let's begin:

1. Come into a position standing on your knees, both partners facing the same direction.

2. Separate from each other so that, when your inside leg is outstretched toward your partner, your toes meet.

3. Slide your inside arm down the inside leg as you arch your torso in toward your partner. Try to keep your body in one plane and let your head be a natural extension of the spine.

4. Extend the outside arm up overhead and in toward your partner. You may or may not be able to reach each other's hands. If you can, place one palm atop the other. Keep your head looking forward and breathe into the rib cage on the outer side of the body.

5. Hold with the arms either stretched overhead or palms touching for five to ten breaths or longer if it is comfortable for both of you. Communicate

When to avoid this posture Do not practice the Perfect Gate if you have a hernia.

Yoga Tip Try this posture by yourself first. Then do it together as described. Notice the differences between going solo and as a team. Which is easier? Which do you prefer?

along the way and encourage each other to breathe and relax.

6. To release, first lift the outside arm and return it back to your side.

7. Use the strength in your abdomen to slide your inner arm back up the leg. Come back to the

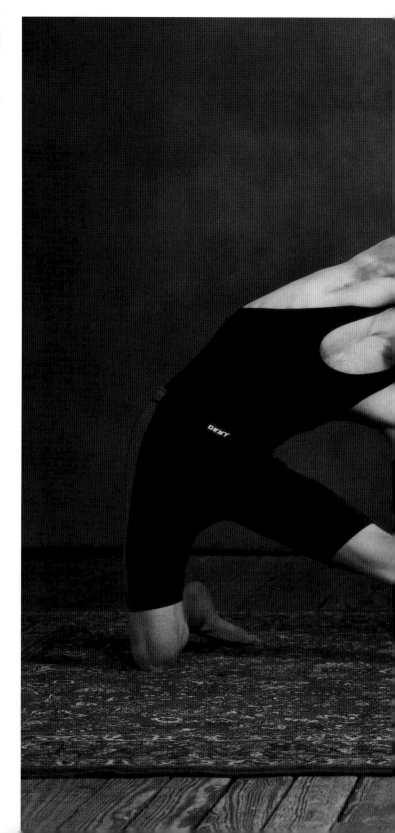

starting kneeling position and do an about-face.

8. Repeat steps 1–7 on the opposite side.

9. When you are done, sit back-to-back with your eyes closed in Proper Sitting Alignment. Connect with your own breath and your partner's breathing rhythm.

No thought, no action, no movement, total stillness: only thus can one manifest the true nature and law of things from within and unconsciously, and at last become one with heaven and earth.

—LAO TZU

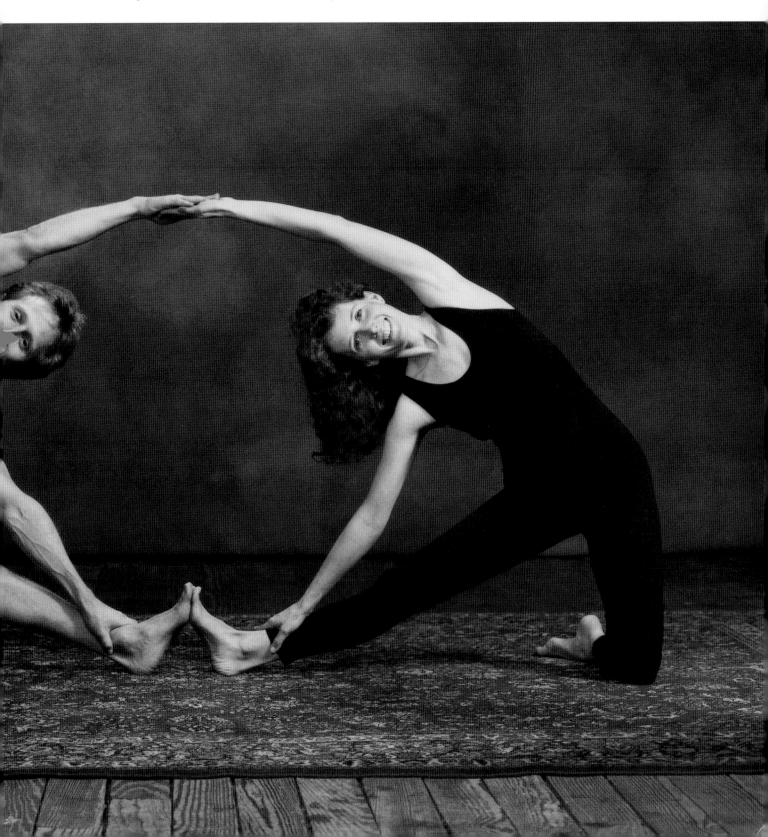

DOUBLE TREE

Benefits:

➤ Improves posture and balance

➤ Focuses and clears mind

➤ Improves concentration

➤ Improves flexibility in ankle, knee, and hip joints

➤ Tones and strengthens legs

➤ Strengthens internal oblique muscles

➤ Improves breathing

Let's begin:

1. Come into Proper Standing Alignment facing the same direction as your partner, as if you are walking down the street together.

2. If you are both about the same height, place the arm closest to each other around your partner's waist. If your partner is significantly taller than you, place your arm around her waist. She can rest her arm around your shoulder.

3. Choose one point on the wall to focus your attention.

4. Both partners: balancing on the inside leg, lift the outside leg and rest the outside foot on either the ankle or knee or up near the groin of the standing leg. Rest your hips against each other.

5. Bring your outside hands together in front of you in prayer position.

6. Don't forget to breathe! Remember to remain lighthearted and explore your balance together with a sense of humor.

7. When you are ready to challenge yourselves further, draw the outside hands up overhead. Either the arms can be directly overhead, or you can attempt to join the palms. Try both positions, although keeping your palms together will be difficult if one of you is significantly taller than the other.

8. Hold the arms overhead for five to ten breaths. If you lose your balance, simply step back in again.

9. To come out of the posture, lower your hands first to prayer position in front of you and then to your sides. Lower the outside leg and turn around to face the opposite wall. Repeat steps 1–9 on the other side.

10. When you are complete, sit back-to-back in Proper Sitting Alignment with your eyes closed for a few breaths.

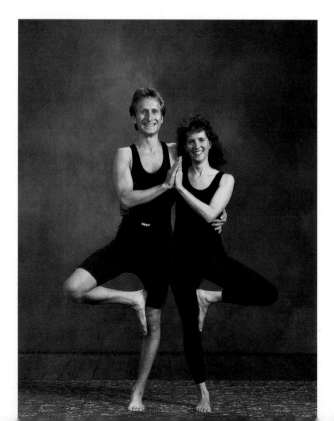

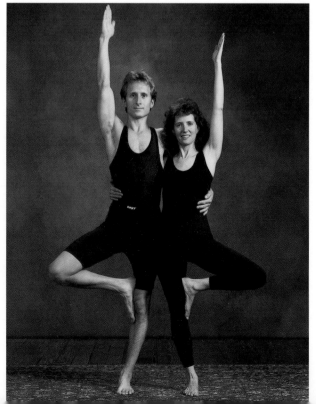

Yoga Tip As you create the Double Tree, consider your roots. Feel your ancestors with you. Consider creating a genealogical tree from both sides of your family. Research the people and stories that brought you to where you are today.

Our band, Five Year Plan, performed tonight. We were great since we all "yogaed" together beforehand and felt totally unified.

—NATALIE CIZMAR, YOGA STUDENT

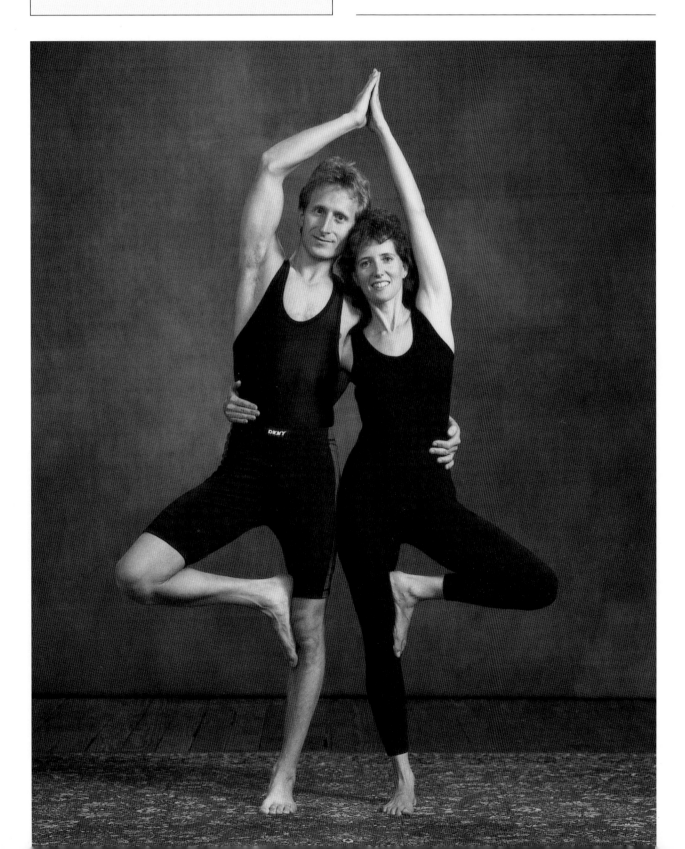

PARTNER PRETZEL TWIST

Body Benefits:

- ➤ Rotates, flexes, extends, tones, and aligns spine
- ➤ Tones abdominals
- ➤ Increases flexibility in the hips
- ➤ Activates digestion and helps relieve constipation
- ➤ Increases circulation
- ➤ Brings fresh oxygen to entire musculo-skeletal system
- ➤ Reduces stiffness in shoulders and neck
- ➤ Strengthens spinal nerves
- ➤ Stimulates liver and spleen

When to avoid this posture Do not practice if you have abdominal hernia.

Yoga Tip As you twist to the first side, imagine you are looking back into your past. As you twist to the opposite side, take a look into your future, seeing visions, hopes, and dreams. When you return to center, sense both polarities and feel yourself connected to the present.

Let's begin:

1. Start in Proper Sitting Alignment facing your partner. Try to touch your bent knees or come as close as you can to each other.

2. Both partners: place your right hand behind you, with the back of the hand against your lower back. Sit up tall.

3. As you face your partner, reach with your left hand over to the right side of your partner's body to clasp the hand behind his or her back. The closer you are the easier it will be.

4. Turn to look away from your partner, over the right shoulder. Press the right shoulder open. Inhale as you lengthen the spine, and exhale more deeply into the twist.

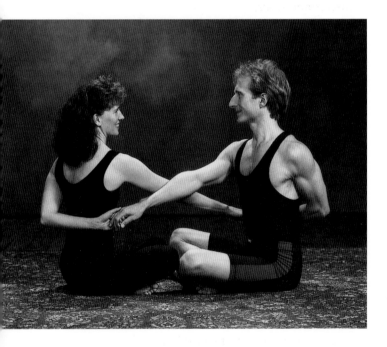

We are like waves that do not move individually but rise and fall in rhythm. To share, to rise and fall in rhythm with life, is a spiritual necessity.

— ALBERT SCHWEITZER

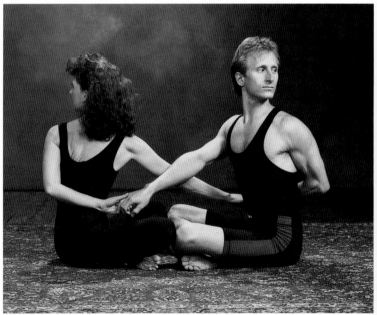

CREATE YOUR OWN POSTURE FOR CONNECTEDNESS

Let's begin:

Part I

1. Complete all of the formal postures before you begin.

2. Come into Proper Standing Alignment facing each other.

3. One of you is the sculptor, the other the clay. Switch after five minutes. You may wish to set a timer.

4. Clay partner: Stand with your eyes closed and take several deep breaths. Feel your connection and trust with your partner. Imagine your body as totally flexible and loose.

5. Sculpting partner: Begin to lightly tap, push, or press a body part of your partner. Clay partner: let your body move naturally in the direction that your partner taps as if you were being directed in a sacred dance.

6. Sculpting partner: You may wish to turn, lower, or lift your partner's shoulders, hips, head, torso, and so on. Be mindful of avoiding parts that are private or ticklish.
   Clay partner: Continue to move, reshape, and dance under your partner's gentle guidance.

7. If at any time either of you feels the clay partner is holding a particularly interesting position, say so. The clay partner can open his eyes and see what he is doing.

8. Switch roles for another five minutes.

Part II

1. After you have both had a turn at being sculptor and clay, you can begin to create a posture that interconnects you in some way. Now you are both clay, and the sculptor is the divine.

2. You may choose to link the same body part or a different one. You may be balanced, twisted, kneeling, back-to-back, or in any other posture you can create to represent your Connectedness. Let your imagination and your bodies explore a multitude of possible interconnections.

3. Hold and breathe when you both find a posture you like and notice how you feel. You may wish to create a statement about your Connectedness that you can affirm during the posture.

4. Once you release, create names for any postures you particularly liked. Take a few minutes to discuss the experience. You may want to create affirmations that represent your Connectedness.

5. For a deeper stretch, lean away from each other.

6. To go even farther into the twist, squeeze your right hand to signal your partner to pull that hand *slowly* toward him or her. This will twist the spine even more, so be sure to let your partner know when to stop.

7. Breathe deeply from your belly all the way up to your throat. Remind your partner to breathe if you suspect that s/he is holding the breath.

8. To release, *slowly* separate hands as if you are in a slow-motion movie. Begin to unwind and return to a comfortable position facing your partner.

9. Repeat steps 1–8, reversing sides.

10. Once you have completed both sides, sit back-to-back with your eyes closed in Proper Sitting Alignment for a few moments. Connect with each other's breath.

INVISIBLE TOUCH MASSAGE

*T*his experience was inspired by Dolores Krieger and Dora Kunz, principal founders of the healing technique known as Therapeutic Touch.

Let's begin:

1. In this experience, you have the opportunity to be both receiver and giver. For a fun way to determine who will be the receiver first, decide who has the shortest hair.

2. Receiver: Come into a comfortable Corpse Pose with your eyes closed. Giver: Sit to one side of your partner.

3. Both partners: Close your eyes and take several long, deep breaths. Come into silence together as a way to connect instantly.

4. Giver: Open your eyes and rub your hands together briskly to generate heat between the palms. Even though your hands won't directly contact the receiver's skin, you will want them to be warm and sensitive. Follow your partner's breath.

5. Giver: Imagine the receiver's body surrounded by an invisible layer that extends two to five inches away from his actual body. This invisible body or energy field is wrinkled. It is your job to smooth it out. As if your hands were irons, begin to press out and smooth out the area, beginning at the head and traveling down to the feet.

6. Giver: Take your time and stay present as you soothe and smooth the invisible body. Sometimes you will be able to find areas that feel hot or cold, tingly, tight, or thick (as if your hands really were in contact with the skin). Some givers may sense various colors, sounds, or other sensory information.

7. Now repeat the entire process from head to toe. In an effort to balance the receiver's energy, go back to areas that you feel require additional attention. For example, if you noticed a cold spot over the abdomen, go back and iron it out with the intention of directing warmth to this area.

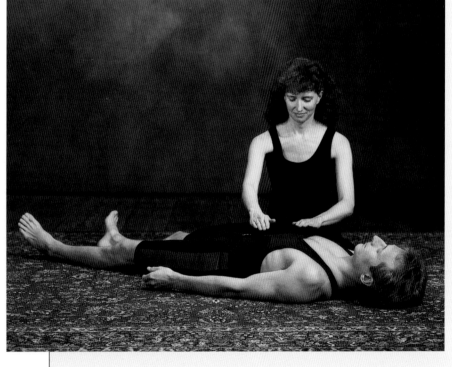

8. This may seem strange at first, but use the creative imagination you had as a child to help you. Imagine that it is your job to evenly distribute a healing blanket over the receiver.

9. When you feel complete, allow your hands to hover over the receiver's body for a moment, wishing your partner well.

10. Without speaking, switch roles.

11. When you have both given and received, spend a few moments quietly sharing about your experiences and any subtle shifts you may have noticed. Thank your partner.

ALPHABETICAL LIST OF POSTURES AND TECHNIQUES

YOGA CENTERS: WHERE TO VISIT AND VACATION

Breitenbush Hot Springs and Retreat
Box 578
Detroit, OR 97342-0578

(503) 854-3314 (leave message, will call back)
E-mail: thebush@teleport.com
Web: www.unotes.com/breitenbush

Canyon Ranch Health Resort
8600 East Rockcliff Road
Tucson, AZ 85750

(800) 726-9900

Coolfont Resort
Cold Run Valley Road, Route 1
Berkeley Springs, WV 25411

(800) 888-8768
E-mail: reservations@coolfont.com

Esalen
Highway 1
Big Sur, CA 93920

(408) 667-3000
Web: www.esalen.org

The Expanding Light
Ananda's Retreat Center
14618 Tyler Foote Road
Nevada City, CA 95959

(800) 346-5350
Web: www.expandinglight.org

Feathered Pipe Ranch
PO Box 1682
Helena, MT 59624

(406) 442-8196
Fax: (406) 442-8110
E-mail: fpranch@ initco.net

The Himalayan Institute
RR 1, Box 400
Honesdale, PA 18431

(800) 822- 4547
E-mail: himalaya@epix.net

Kripalu Center for Yoga and Health
Box 793
Lenox, MA 01240

(800) 741-SELF (7353)
Fax: (413) 448-3196
Web: www.kripalu.org

Mohonk Mountain Retreat
Lake Mohonk
New Paltz, NY 12561

(800) 772-6646

Mount Madonna Center
445 Summit Road
Watsonville, CA 95076

(408) 847-0406
E-mail: Programs@MountMadonna.org
Web: www.infopoint.com/orgs/mmc

Norwich Inn & Spa
607 West Thames (Route 32)
Norwich, CT 06360

(800) ASK-4SPA

Omega Institute for Holistic Studies
260 Lake Drive
Rhinebeck, NY 12572

(800) 944-1001
E-mail: info@omega-inst.org
Web: www.omega-inst.org

Satchidananda Ashram—Yogaville
Route 1 Box 1720
Buckingham, VA 23921

(800) 858-YOGA

Sivananda Ashram Yoga Ranch Colony
PO Box 195, Budd Road
Woodbourne, NY 12788

(914) 434-9242
E-mail: YogaRanch@sivananda.org

For information about other locations including Paradise Island, Bahamas; Val Morin, Quebec; Grass Valley, CA; and Kerala, India, call: (800) 783-YOGA, or Web: www.sivananda.org

ABOUT THE MODELS

Stephen Cope (Focus and Compassion) is a program director and scholar-in-residence at Kripalu Center for Yoga and Health, where he spent 1995 through 1997 working on a book about the psychology of the eight-stage path of yoga (Bantam, 1998, as yet untitled). He finds that his yoga practice deeply supports his writing because, as he says, "When I'm writing well, the words seem to flow from my body, not my mind." He is also a cyclist and a classical pianist.

Elly Gardner (Energy and Balance) incorporates yoga into her occupational therapy practice with children. She is eternally grateful to her yoga teachers and students. She enjoys movies, dancing, and talking with her friends.

Ann Greene (Connectedness) and her husband, Todd Norian, coteach Kripalu Yoga Teacher Training as well as Partner Yoga. Together they enjoy hiking, biking, running, and skiing. Ann also teaches yoga at Canyon Ranch in the Berkshires. She uses yoga as a tool of support through life's transitions.

Juliarose Loffredo (Peace and Playfulness) is one of Rachel's yoga students. She is a weaver/dyer/fiber artist. She often sits with her legs in the Hero Pose (which is her favorite yoga posture) when she designs and sews her work. She collects other people's junk and creates art with it. She enjoys being silly, walking around barefoot, and macaroni and cheese.

Ian Magpantay (Awareness and Confidence) is one of Rachel's yoga students. Yoga brought him to a deeper level of Awareness of how to take better care of his mind and body. Ian has a sincere fascination with life and the sciences. He loves surfing and hopes to surf the world. His dream is to return someday to his birthplace in the Philippines.

Todd Norian (Connectedness) has a passion for yoga and meditation. He has trained over one thousand teachers at Kripalu Center and is a Phoenix Rising Yoga Therapist. He teaches workshops throughout the country and works with private clients. He is an accomplished musician and has produced music for yoga and relaxation.

Alicia Scott (Strength and Acceptance) is one of Rachel's yoga students. When she started taking yoga she was extremely shy. She is now self-assured, forthright, and eager. She plans to become a yoga teacher herself as well as a therapist. She wakes up at 5:00 A.M. daily to practice yoga, as it helps to deepen her prayer life. She loves to read, to spend time with children, and to take bubble baths.

Madeleine Weinrich (Flexibility) lives with her husband, Roger, and two sons, Adam and Max, in an antique farmhouse in the woods. She owns and operates a really cool consignment shop called Good Fortune in Keene, New Hampshire. She also teaches yoga workshops throughout the United States and Canada. Through her daily yoga practice, she maintains Flexibility in both her body and her busy life.

ABOUT THE PHOTOGRAPHERS

Adam Mastoon and **David S. Waitz** have been friends for more than sixteen years. They studied photography together in New York and Paris. This is their first collaborative work. Each pursues his own photographic career. Mastoon is a social documentarian and portrait photographer currently residing in Lenox Massachusetts. His work has appeared in numerous publications. His first book of portraits entitled *The Shared Heart* was published by William Morrow and Co. in 1997. Waitz is a digital photographic illustrator living in New York City. He creates images for both advertising and editorial clients.

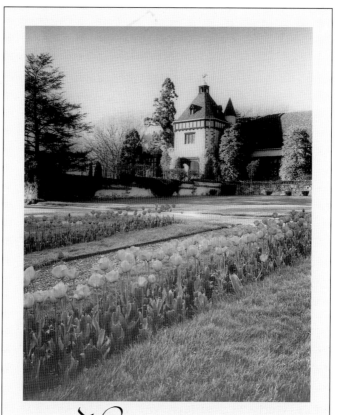

Many of the photographs for
Yoga for Your Spiritual Muscles were taken at the
famed Pleasantdale Chateau and Conference
Resort. Located on a secluded forty-acre estate in
West Orange, New Jersey, Pleasantdale offers
state-of-the-art meeting facilities as well as
antique-appointed overnight accomodations and
special party rooms. Its formal gardens, rolling
lawns, shaded ponds, and woodlands provided an
exquisite and tranquil backdrop for yoga.

QUEST BOOKS
are published by
The Theosophical Society in America,
Wheaton, Illinois 60189-0270,
a branch of a world organization
dedicated to the promotion of the unity of
humanity and the encouragement of the study of
religion, philosophy, and science, to the end that
we may better understand ourselves and our place in
the universe. The Society stands for complete
freedom of individual search and belief.
For further information about its activities,
write, call 1-800-669-1571, or consult its Web page:
http://www.theosophical.org

The Theosophical Publishing House
is aided by the generous support of
THE KERN FOUNDATION,
a trust established by Herbert A. Kern
and dedicated to Theosophical education.